The I

By Charles A. Tyrrell, M.D.

PREFACE

TO THE ONE HUNDREDTH EDITION.

In presenting to the public the one hundredth edition of this work, it is a matter for profound gratification to be able to state that the treatment described in its pages has steadily increased in public favor since its introduction. Tens of thousands of grateful people testify to its efficiency, not only as a remedial process, but better still, as a preventive of disease. Truth must ever prevail, and this treatment being based on natural law (which is unerring), must achieve the desired result, which is the restoration and preservation of health.

This edition has been completely revised and much of it rewritten, and, while the essential principles remain unchanged, some slight departures from previously expressed opinions may be noted; for in the years that have elapsed since the first edition saw the light, some notable advances have been made in rational therapeutics and dietetics, and no one can afford to lag behind the car of Progress.

The arrangement of the book has been still farther altered, by adding another part, making nine in all, each part being devoted to a special phase of the general subject, thus simplifying it, and making its principles easier of application. Quotations have been freely made from articles written during the past three years by the author, in his capacity as editor of "Health," and several new formulas for the treatment of important diseases have been added to those that have appeared in previous editions.

While painfully conscious that the critically disposed may find something to condemn in its pages, the work is sent forth with the fervent hope, that despite any defects it may possess it may, in the future, as in the past, prove the means of restoring to suffering thousands the possession of their natural and rightful heritage health.

THE AUTHOR.

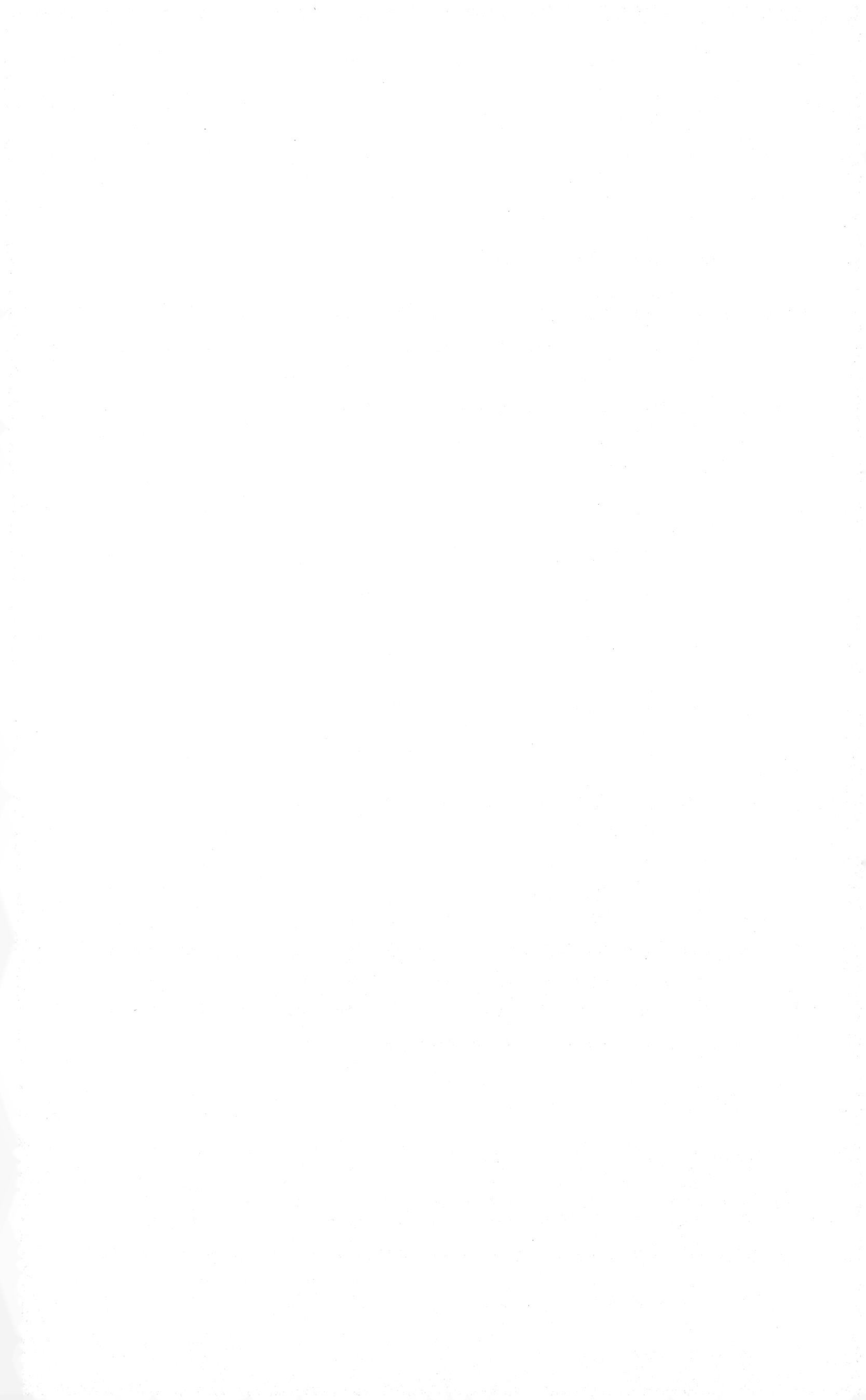

CONTENTS.

treatment.

PART V.

PRACTICAL HYGIENE.

Longevity man's natural heritage. The care of the body absolute cleanliness rare. The function of water in the human organism. Hot water the natural scavenger. The bath. Description of the skin, and its function. Hints on bathing. The wet sheet pack. Importance of fresh air. Interchange of gases in the lungs. Ventilation. Prof. Willard Parker on impure air. The function of the heart. The therapeutic value of sunlight.

PART VI.

EXERCISE.

Motion is life. Effect of exercise on the fluids of the body. How the tissues are nourished. Exercise for invalids. Complete system of breathing exercises for developing the lungs. Improved system of physical exercises, calling into play every muscle of the body ensuring harmonious development. Special nerve exercise. how to stand and how to walk. All the above exercises plainly illustrated.

PART VII.

THE DIET QUESTION.

The replacement of waste. Appetite and hunger. The evils of gluttony. Vegetarianism versus flesh eating. Diet, a question of latitude. The cause of old age. Cretinism. Danger of earthy matters in food substances. Fruits are ideal foods. The true value of bread. Classification of the ingredients of food substances. Table of proportions. Table of digestive values. Vegetarianism discussed. A mixed diet the most reasonable. How to eat. Liquids at meals. When to eat. The no breakfast plan. The effects of alcohol, tea and coffee. Improper habits of eating. The influence of mind upon digestion. The advantages of regularity. Nature's bookkeeping.

PART VIII.

TREATMENT OF DISEASE.

Complete formulas of treatment (with dietary rules) for over fifty different diseases, including Consumption, Appendicitis, Locomotor Ataxia, Paralysis, Dyspepsia, Pneumonia, Diabetes Mellitus, Uterine troubles, etc. Also all the principal ailments of children.

PART IX.

SOME HELPFUL SUGGESTIONS.

Disease is the result of the operation of natural law don't dread it. Don't treat symptoms; treat the fundamental cause. Pain is Nature's danger signal. Prevention is better than cure. The elements of prevention. Importance of a knowledge of physiology. The body, the vehicle of expression for the mind. The strenuous life. Tear worse than wear. The importance of reserve energy. The effect of the mind on the body. The human body as a bank. The importance of a daily balance. Cultivate cheerfulness. The habit of happiness. The folly of squandering health. Medicine and surgery compared. What children should be taught. The final word.

APPENDIX.

Instructions for massage. How to use the stomach bath by three different methods. How to improvise the Turkish Bath in your own home, without apparatus. How to use the wet sheet pack. How to care for the "Cascade".

THE ROYAL ROAD TO HEALTH.

PART I.

DRUGGING PROVED UNSCIENTIFIC.

It is one of the most profound mysteries of our civilization, and has been one of the most perplexing and discouraging phenomena of human existence, that, while the world at large has maintained an ever increasing "medical profession," whose members are popularly supposed to be competent to deal with all the ills that flesh is heir to; still there has always been a long list of what are termed "incurable diseases." But the immense strides made, in recent years, in every branch of modern science, has led the thinking public to consider such a condition of things as an outrageous libel on the God of Nature, and to question whether there can be such a thing as an incurable disease.

Health is such an inestimable blessing, that the individual who shall devise means to preserve it, or to restore it, when lost, is deserving of all the thanks and honors that a grateful community can bestow. Unfortunately, there are very few who estimate life at its true value, until they are confronted with the grim destroyer, Death. No one can fully appreciate the priceless blessings of health, until they feel that it has slipped from their grasp. The oft quoted phrase, "Health is Wealth," is truly a concrete expression of wisdom, for without the former, the latter is well nigh an impossibility. But its interference with the activities of life is one of the least evils of sickness, for perfect health is the very salt and spice of life; without it, existence is "weary, stale, flat and unprofitable."

But let none despair, for it is my purpose to show how those who enjoy the blessing of robust health may preserve it indefinitely, and how those who have lost it may regain it with access of vigor, and once more feel that life is indeed worth living. In presenting a new system of medication, it is necessary to attack the existing systems, and hence, I am placed in a delicate position, for of all the problems ever presented for the ingenuity of man to solve, undoubtedly the most difficult is, how to present new facts so as not to offend old errors; for individuals are very prone to regard arguments levelled against their opinions as direct attacks upon their personality; and not a few of them mistake their own deeply rooted prejudices for established certainties.

I shall endeavor to show that the practice of administering drugs to cure disease is a fallacy, and in so doing, I am bound to incur the condemnation of my brother practitioners, who prescribe drugs, and the druggists who vend them.

It may safely be asserted that the drug system of treating disease would be destroyed if it were to be critically examined; in fact, to defend it is provocative of unmistakable damage to it. If it is once subjected to the analysis of calm reason its defects become palpable to the meanest understanding.

There are three principal schools of medicine, each with a distinctive title, but they are all one in essential principles. They may differ in unimportant details; but in the main premises they are a unit. They all believe in the principle of "curing one disease by producing another." In other words, their practice is, to induce a drug disease to cure a primary one, for this is exactly what is done when drugs are administered, in pathological conditions as we shall prove later on by testimony from authorities on medical practice.

The materia medica of the schools, to-day, includes upwards of two thousand substances the number increasing daily and when viewed dispassionately it presents what? A list of drugs, chemicals, dye- stuffs, all subversive of organic structures. They are all antagonistic to living matter: all produce disease when brought in contact in any manner with the living domain as a matter of fact, all are poisons. Now, what logical standing can a system have, that employs, as remedies for diseases, those things that produce disease in healthy persons? No advocate of the drug system has ever advanced a reason that would bear one moment's scientific examination, why poisonous substances should be administered to the sick, and no one will ever be able to give a satisfactory explanation of the theory that underlies the practice, for none exists. When once the public fully grasps the true import of this glaring anomaly, the days of the drug system will be numbered.

Physicians of ability and long experience, who have devoted their lives to the relief of suffering humanity, both in this and other countries, have declared after close observation, that they were fully and thoroughly convinced that medicines do not cure patients, that they do not assist Nature's process of cure, so much as they retard it, and, that they are more hurtful than remedial in all diseases. A still larger number have reached the same conclusion with regard to certain complaints, such as scarlet fever, croup, pneumonia, cholera, rheumatism, diphtheria, measles, small-pox, dysentery, and typhoid fever, and that in every case where they have abandoned all medicine, abjured all drugs and potions, their success has been marvellously increased.

Professor B. F. Parker, of the New York Medical College, once said to a medical class: "I have recently given no medicine in the treatment of measles and scarlet fever, and I have had excellent success."

Dr. Snow, Health Officer of Providence, R. I., reported for the information of his professional brethren, through the Boston Medical and Surgical Journal that he had treated all the cases of small-pox, which had prevailed endemically in that city, without a particle of medicine, and that all of the cases some of which were very grave ones recovered.

Dr. John Bell, Professor of Materia Medica in one of the Philadelphia Colleges, and also in the Medical College of Baltimore, testified in a work which he published ("Bell on Baths"), that he and others had treated many cases of scarlet fever with bathing, and without medicines of any kind, and without losing a patient.

Dr. Ames, of Montgomery, Alabama, some years since published in the New Orleans Medical and Surgical Journal, his experience and observation in the treatment of pneumonia. He had been led to notice for many years, that patients who were treated with the ordinary remedies--bleeding, mercury, and remedies--breeding certain complications which always aggravated the malady, and rendered the convalescence more lingering and recovery less complete. Such patients were always liable to collapses and re-lapses; to "run into typhoid"; to sink suddenly, and die very unexpectedly.

He noticed particularly that patients who took calomel and antimony were found, on post-mortem examinations, to have serious and even fatal inflammation of the stomach and small intestines, attended with great prostration, delirium, and other symptoms of drug poisoning. These "complications" were nothing more or less than drug diseases. And Dr. Ames found, on changing his plan of treatment to milder and simpler remedies, that he lost no patients.

The late Professor Win. Tully, M.D., of Yale College, and of the Vermont Academy of Medicine at Gastleton, Vt., informed his medical class, that on one occasion the typhoid pneumonia was so fatal in some places in the valley of the Connecticut River, that the people became suspicious that the physicians were doing more harm than good; and in their desperation they actually combined against the doctors and refused to employ them at all; "after which," said Professor Tully, "no deaths occurred." And I might add, as an historical incident of some pertinency in this place, that regular physicians were once banished from Rome, so fatal did their practice seem, so far as the people could judge of it.

The great Magendie, of France, who long stood at the very head of Physiology and Pathology in the French Academy which, by the way, has claimed to be, and perhaps is, the most learned body of men in the world performed this experiment. He divided the patients of one of the large Paris hospitals into three classes. To one he prescribed the common remedies of the books. To the second he administered only the common simples of domestic practice. And to the third class he gave no medicine at all. The result was, those who took less medicine did better than those who took more, and those who took no medicine did the best of all.

Magendie also divided his typhoid fever patients into two classes, to one of whom he prescribed the ordinary remedies, and to the other no medicines at all, relying wholly on such nursing and such attention to Hygiene as the vital instincts demanded and common sense suggested. Of the patients who were treated the usual way, he lost the usual proportion, about one-fourth. And of those who took no medicine, he lost none. And what opinion has Magendie left on record of the popular healing art? He said to his medical class, "Gentlemen, medicine is a great humbug."

In the face of such damaging testimony from prominent representatives of the medical profession, it becomes exceedingly difficult to place any reliance on the drug remedies prescribed by them.

The melancholy truth is, that drug medication has become an integral part of our domestic economy. At no time in history has the consumption of drugs even approximated the present rate. Enormous sums of money are invested in manufacturing and distributing them, and the physicians of the various schools, being educated to prescribe them, a mutual bond of interest has grown up between doctor and druggist, which is not at all surprising. The medical profession, as a whole is, and ever has been eminently conservative, and this fact, in connection with its traditional predilection for drugs causes its members to resolutely set their faces against any remedial process that runs counter to the theories they imbibed at college. They look askance at all such things and regard them as dangerous experiments, and assert that their dignity will not permit them to recognize any irregular practice, or any form of quackery.

Dignity! When was dignity ever known to save a life? Most humanity continue to suffer because the medical profession (blindly following in the rut of custom) fail to see anything superior to the antiquated system of treating disease by drugging, which many of its ablest members condemn as unreliable?

It is with all schools of medicine as it is with each individual practitioner of the healing art the less faith they have in medicine, the more they have in Hygiene; hence those who prescribe little or no medicine, are invariably and necessarily more attentive to Hygiene, which always was, and ever will be, all that there is really good, useful, or curative in medication. Such physicians are more careful to supply the vital organism with whatever of air, light, temperature, food, water, exercise or rest, etc., it needs in its struggle for health, and to remove all vitiating influences all poisons, impurities, or disturbing influences of any kind. This is hygienic medication, the natural and rational method of cure, and the more closely it is examined, the more strongly it will commend itself to reason.

It is a lamentable fact that the preservation of health is not taught in the medical schools, neither is it explained in their books, and judging from general practice not much regard is attached to it in their prescriptions. But when the inevitable typhoid or malaria appears as an inevitable consequence of neglected precautions, the physician can drug without mercy, and, as we contend, on most illogical grounds.

Who imagines for one instant, that quinine is a poison? Who is not aware that arsenic is a deadly poison? And yet physicians and medical journals calmly and gravely assert that arsenic is the better article of the two, and recommend it as a substitute for quinine. Can any intelligent person believe that a comparatively harmless tonic, and an intense poison are perfect equivalents for each other?

It is stated on reliable authority, that during the civil war, hundreds of sick soldiers implored the nurses to throw away their medicine. They feared drugs worse than bullets, and not without reason.

It is a curious fact that young physicians prescribe more medicine than the older ones.

Said the venerable Professor Alexander H. Stevens M.D., of the New York College of Physicians and Surgeons: "Young practitioners are a most hopeful class of community. They are sure of success. They start out in life with twenty remedies for every disease; and after an experience of thirty years or less they find twenty diseases for every remedy." And again: "The older physicians grow, the more skeptical they become of the virtues of medicine, and the more they are disposed to trust to the powers of Nature."

The effect of drugging a person, is to lock up the actual causes of the disease in the system; thus producing permanent and worse diseases. It is in accordance with common sense that they should be expelled, not retained. What is known as disease, is nothing more or less than the struggle of Nature, to cast out impurities, and this remedial effort should be regulated, and assisted, not obstructed by administering drugs, which only complicate the situation, by producing more disease.

No man can fight two enemies better than one, and, to give drugs to a system already struggling to regain its normal condition, is like tying the hands of a man who is beset by enemies. The truth is, that the real nature of disease is misapprehended by the popular schools of medicine, and until broader views obtain a lodgment among them, it is useless to hope for any alteration or improvement in the antiquated system of drugging. "Who shall decide, when doctors disagree ?" is an oft Quoted sentence, and, the following conflicting opinions from prominent physicians show conclusively how little is actually known of the action of drugs upon the human system, by those who administer them right and left.

Says the "United States Dispensatory," "Medicines are those articles which make sanative impressions on the body." This may be important if, true. But, per contra, says Professor Martin Paine, M.D., of the New York University Medical School, in his "Institutes of Medicine": "Remedial agents are essentially morbific in their operations."

But again says Professor Paine: "Remedial agents operate in the same manner as do the remote causes of disease." This seems to be a very distinct announcement that remedies are themselves causes of disease. And yet again: "In the administration of medicines we cure one disease by producing another." This is both important and true.

Professor Paine quotes approvingly the famous professional adage, in good technical Latin,

"Ubi virus, ibi vitus,"

which, being translated, means, "our strongest poisons are our best remedies."

Says Professor Alonzo Clark, M.D., of the New York College of Physicians and Surgeons: "All of our curative agents are poisons, and as a consequence, every dose diminishes the patient's vitality."

Says Professor Joseph M. Smith, M.D., of the same school: "All medicines which enter the circulation poison the blood in the same manner as do the poisons that produce disease."

Says Professor St. John, of the New York Medical College : "All medicines are poisonous."

Says Professor B. R. Peaslee, MD., of the same school: "The administration of powerful medicines is the most fruitful cause of derangements of the digestion."

Says Professor H. G. Cox, M.D., of the same school: "The fewer remedies you employ in any disease, the better for your patients."

Says Professor E. H. Davis, M.D., of the New York Medical College: "The modus operandi of medicines is still a very obscure subject. We know that they operate, but exactly how they operate is entirely unknown."

Says Professor J. W. Carson, M.D., of the New York University Medical School: "We do not know whether our patients recover because we give medicines, or because Nature cures them."

Says Professor E. S. Carr, of the same school: "All drugs are more or less adulterated; and as not more than one physician in a hundred has sufficient knowledge in chemistry to detect impurities, the physician seldom knows just how much of a remedy he is prescribing."

The authors disagree in many things; but all concur in the fact that medicines produce diseases; that their effects are wholly uncertain, and that we know nothing whatever of their modus operandi.

But now comes in the testimony of the venerable Professor Joseph M. Smith, M.D., who says: "Drugs do not cure diseases; disease is always cured by the vis medicatrix naturae."

And Professor Clark further complicates the problem before us by declaring that, "Physicians have hurried thousands to their graves who would have recovered if left to Nature." And again: "In scarlet fever you have nothing to do but to rely on the vis medicatrix naturae."

Says Professor Gross: "Of the essence of disease very little is known; indeed, nothing at all." And says Professor George B. Wood, M.D., of Jefferson Medical College, Philadelphia ("Wood's Practice of Medicine"): "Efforts have been made to reach the elements of disease; but not very successfully; because we have not yet learned the essential nature of the healthy actions, and cannot understand their derangements."

On the other side of the Atlantic the claims of the existing medical schools to popular favor, do not appear to rest upon any surer basis than they do here, if we may judge from the following opinions expressed by some of the most eminent authorities in the British Kingdom:

"The medical practice of our days is, at the best, a most uncertain and unsatisfactory system; it has neither philosophy nor common sense to commend it to confidence." DR. EVANS, Fellow of the Royal College, London.

"There has been a great increase of medical men of late, but, upon my life, diseases have increased in proportion." JOHN ABERNETHY, M.D., "The Good," of London.

"Gentlemen, ninety-nine out of every hundred medical facts are medical lies; and medical doctrines are, for the most part, stark, staring nonsense." Prof. GREGORY, of Edinburgh, author of a work on "Theory and Practice of Physic."

"It cannot be denied that the present system of medicine is a burning shame to its professors, if indeed a series of vague and uncertain incongruities deserves to be called by that name. How rarely do our medicines do good! How often do they make our patients really worse! I fearlessly assert, that in most cases the sufferer would be safer without a physician than with one. I have seen enough of the malpractice of my professional. brethren to warrant the strong language I employ." Dr. RAMAGE, Fellow of the Royal College, London.

"The present practice of medicine is a reproach to the name of Science, while its professors give evidence of an almost total ignorance of the nature and proper treatment of disease. Nine times out of ten, our miscalled remedies are absolutely injurious to our patients, suffering under diseases of whose real character and cause we are most culpably ignorant." Prof. JAMEISON, of Edinburgh.

Assuredly the uncertain and most unsatisfactory art that we call medical science, is no science at all, but a jumble of inconsistent opinions; of conclusions hastily and often incorrectly drawn; of facts misunderstood or perverted; of comparisons without analogy; of hypotheses without reason, and theories not only useless, but dangerous." Dublin Medical Journal.

"Some patients get well with the aid of medicine; more without it; and still more in spite of it." SIR JOHN FORBES, M.D., F.R.S.

"Thousands are annually slaughtered in the quiet of the sick-room.' Governments should at once either banish medical men, and proscribe their blundering art, or they should adopt some better means to protect the lives of the people than at present prevail, when they look far less after the practice of this dangerous profession, and the murders committed in it, than after the lowest trades." Dr FRANK, an eminent author and practitioner.

"Our actual information or knowledge of disease does not increase in proportion to our experimental practice. Every dose of medicine given is a blind experiment upon the vitality of the patient." Dr. BOSTOCK, author of "History of Medicine."

"The science of medicine is a barbarous jargon, and the effects of our medicines on the human system in the highest degree uncertain; except, indeed, that they have destroyed more lives than war, pestilence, and famine combined." JOHN MASON GOOD, M.D., F.R.S., author of "Book of Nature," "A System of Nosology," "Study of Medicine," etc.

"I declare as my conscientious conviction, founded on long experience and reflection, that if there were not a single physician, surgeon, man midwife, chemist, apothecary, druggist, nor drug on the face of the earth, there would be less sickness and less mortality than now prevail." JAS. JOHNSON, M.D., F.R.S., Editor of the Medico- Chirurgical Review.

So it comes to this, that during three thousand years remedies have been accumulating until between two and three thousand drugs are recorded in the archives of the medical profession, and yet we have the admission of some of the highest authorities on the subject that the nature of disease is still a mystery, that the "modus operandi" of drugs is equally obscure, and that in consequence there is profound uncertainty as to the relation of drugs to the diseases for which they are prescribed.

Can one cause cure another. Can a poison expel a poison? Can the human system throw off two burdens better than one? If such a proposition were submitted to us in any other domain we would indignantly resent it as an insult to our intelligence.

There can be no question but that the public are largely responsible for the existing condition of things, for whatever they demand they can obtain, in obedience to the inexorable law of supply and demand: which accounts for the rapidly increasing interest in hygiene. An eminent authority on therapeutics says:

"The medical profession holds a most false relation to society. Its honors and emoluments are measured, not by the good, but by the evil it does. The physician who keeps some member of the family of his rich neighbor on a bed of sickness for months or years, may secure to himself thereby both fame and fortune; while the other who would restore the patient to health in a week or two, will be neither appreciated nor understood. If a physician, in treating a simple fever, which if left to itself or to Nature would terminate in health in two or three weeks, drugs the patient into half a dozen chronic diseases, and nearly kills himself half a dozen times, and prolongs his sufferings for months, he will receive much money and many thanks for carrying him safely through so many complications, relapses, and collapses. But if he cures in a single week, and leaves him perfectly sound, the pay will be small, and the thanks nowhere, because he has not been very sick!

"I know many of you will say, 'My physician is a very excellent man and a good scholar I have all confidence in him.' But what if his system is false? Is your confidence in him or in his system? If in his system, you are to be pitied. If in him, take his good advice and refuse his bad medicine."

The Caucasian has not much to learn from the Mongolian, it is true, but the public might safely imitate the Chinese in dealing with their physicians. A Chinaman of rank pays his physician a retaining salary so long as he remains in health, but, the instant he gets sick, the salary ceases. Manifestly, it is a common sense proceeding. The doctor has a vital interest in preserving the health of his client, since sickness entails a pecuniary loss; and best of all, the patient escapes having his system drenched with drugs. There is no valid reason why there should be any such thing as serious sickness; nor would there be if Hygiene were taught, and practised, and the whole materia medica consigned to oblivion. As Dr. Oliver Wendell Holmes said, "If all drugs were thrown into the sea, it would be so much better for man, but so much worse for the fishes."

Now, the remedies of the Hygienic system, which I advocate, comprehend everything except poisons. The drug system rejects almost everything but poisons. My system rejects only poisons, and adopts everything else. I welcome anything that possesses remedial value, provided it is in accordance with the laws of Nature, and am equally ready to accept suggestions from the laity, as from fellow practitioners. I am ready to submit everything thus presented, to the test of experiment, and employ it if found worthy.

In this regard I may, without vanity, lay claim to the possession of a more progressive spirit than the members of the drug schools, for their disincilination to adopt anything new in the treatment of disease has passed into a proverb. It might naturally be supposed that any one who should come forward with a discovery by which the suffering portion. of the human family would be benefited, would be welcomed with open arms by the medical fraternity, or, that at least he would be allowed a hearing, but unfortunately it is not so.

Even if the discoverer be one of themselves, they are apt to regard his proposition with a certain amount of distrust, but if he happens to be a layman they instantly stand upon their dignity denounce all irregular practice and raise the cry of quack.

In justice, however, it must be said that there are members of liberal, broad minded men in the medical profession who recognize the fact that brains are not monopolized by physicians, and who are perfectly willing to accord credit where it is due, as the following opinions will show.

Dr. A. O'Leary, Jefferson Medical College, of Philadelphia, says:

"The best things in the healing art have been done by those who never had a diploma the first Caesarian section, lithotomy, the use of cinchona, of ether as an anaesthetic, the treatment of the air passages by inhalation, the water cure and medicated baths, electricity as a healing agent, and magnetism, faith cure, mind cure, etc."

Prof. Waterhouse, writing to the learned Dr. Mitchell, of New York, says:

"I am, indeed, so disgusted with learned quackery that I take some interest in honest, humane, and strongminded empiricism; for it has done more for our art, in all ages and all countries, than all the universities since the time of Charlemagne."

Professor Benj. Rush, of the greatest and oldest Allopathic College in America, says:

"Remember how many of our most useful remedies have been discovered by quacks. Do not therefore be afraid of conversing with them, and of profiting by their ignorance and temerity. Medicine has its pharisees as well as religion. But the spirit of this sect is as unfriendly to the advancement of medicine as it is to Christian charity. In the pursuit of medical knowledge let me advise you to converse with nurses and old women. They will often suggest facts in the history and cure of disease which have escaped the most sagacious observers of nature. By so doing, we may discover laws of the animal economy which have no place in our system of Nosology, or in our theories of physic. The practice of physic hath been more improved by the casual experiments of illiterate nations, and the rash ones of vagabond quacks, than by all the once celebrated professors of it, and the theoretic teachers in the several schools of Europe, very few of whom have furnished us with one new medicine, or have taught us better to use our old ones, or have in any one instance at all, improved the art of curing disease."

Dr. Adam Smith says:

"After denouncing Paracelsus as a quack, the regular medical profession stole his `quack-silver' mercury; after calling Jenner an imposter it adopted his discovery of vaccination; after dubbing Harvey a humbug it was forced to swallow his theory of the circulation of the blood."

Professor J. Rodes Buchanan, Boston, says:

"Mozart, Hoffman, Ole Bull, and Blind Tom were born with a mastery of music, as Zerah Colburn with a mastery of mathematics, as others are born with a mastery of the mystery of life and disease, like Greatrakes, Newton, Hutton, Sweet and Stephens, born doctors, and score of similar renown."

Professor Charles W. Emerson, M.D., the well known resident of the Monroe Conservatory of Oratory, of Boston, says:

"The progress in therapeutics has and still continues to come from the unlearned. Common people give us our improvements and the school men spend their time in giving Greek and Latin names to these improvements, and building metaphysical theories around them."

This is a heavy indictment against the medical profession, as a body, but truth and justice compel me to state that most of the foregoing statements were made some years ago, and that intolerance can no longer be charged against them as it could, even in the last generation. Nor can we close our eyes to the fact that thousands of highminded physicians are devoting their time and energies to the amelioration of disease. Scarcely a month passes in which some convention of physicians is not held to consider the best means of dealing with some particular malady, and a large number of the attending physicians at those conventions contribute their time and experience at considerable financial loss to themselves.

In the ranks of the medical body there are able and honorable men who would adorn any profession--men who have sacrificed health, wealth and happiness in their devotion to the cause of suffering humanity the pages of history are full of instances of such heroism. But of what avail is it to have the most perfect examples of humanity for physicians, if the system they practice is an erroneous one? It is impossible to secure good results with bad methods. We must have a sure foundation, if we expect to raise an abiding structure. And that is why I am in opposition to the existing method of treating disease. Not because of any feeling against the physician individually, but for the reason that I consider their system based upon error upon a false conception of the true nature of disease, and of the relation of drugs to the human system.

There is a tradition in the orthodox medical schools, that all curative processes are dependent upon, and act only in accordance With, an established law the "Law of Cure."

But although all the schools are a unit in believing in the existence and operation of such a law, no two of them agree upon a definition of it. Their theories concerning this all important law are as diametrically opposite as the poles. For instance, the Allopaths define it as "contraria contrariis curantur," which is simply the law of opposition. But the Homeopaths take a widely different view of the matter, their definition of it being "similia similibus curantur," which is, practically, the law of agreement; while the Eclectics declare that "sanative medication" is the law.

This diversity of opinion is not by any means unique, for the tendency to disagreement among physicians is proverbial; but the unfortunate layman who is the person most vitally interested in the matter, is at a loss what to believe among this conflict of definitions, and naturally asks, Who is right?

I answer, unequivocally, not one! They are all wrong. This so-called "Law of Cure" is a purely imaginary affair; one of the many misconceptions peculiar to the medical schools, originating in a false conception of the true nature of disease. There is no such thing as a law of cure! There is a condition of cure, and that is, obedience. Nature has provided penalties for disobedience, and is inexorable in exacting payment; but she does not provide remedies. If there is one thing absolutely certain in nature, it is the unfaltering sequence of cause and effect. Nature never stultifies herself. It is impossible to imagine nature providing penalties for violation of her laws, and then furnishing remedies to make those penalties negatory.

It is a lamentable fact that the medical profession, as a body, entertain a totally erroneous conception of the true nature of disease, and its legitimate function in the economy of nature. Instead of recognizing it as a beneficent remedial process, which, if properly aided, will work out the salvation of the patient, they antagonize it at every turn, and endeavor to suppress the symptoms, which are its legitimate expressions.

The whole thing is a huge misconception, the failure to understand the true relation between living and dead substances. According to the United States Dispensatory, medicines are those substances That make sanative impressions on the body.

A false definition of a word leads to a false system of remedial practice, based upon that definition. What is an impression? Is it the action of a dead substance, which cannot act upon a living substance that can? Assuredly not! Is it not rather the recognition by the living substance of the lifeless one? The whole theory of drug action is easily explainable on this hypothesis. Drugs--inert substances--do not act upon the living organism, but are acted upon, with a view to their expulsion from the living domain. If it were not so, if drugs really acted upon the various organs, then their action should be equally as effective after death as before. But no, nature resents the introduction of foreign substances into the human economy, and exerts all her powers to cast out the intruders.

Now, as all substances incapable of physiological use are foreign, such as particles of worn out tissue, the waste products of digestion, etc., and their presence in the animal economy inimical to the general welfare, the depurating organs are called into active play to expel the offending substances; and the increased physiological activity, and (in the case of actual lesion) the increased flow of blood to the parts, for the purpose of repair, cause a rise in temperature, commonly known as fever, which is one of the most frequent symptoms of what is generally recognized as disease; thus establishing the fact, indisputably, that disease is purely and simply a remedial process, either for purposes of repair or purification.

The practice, therefore, of increasing the deposits in the physical system by the introduction of drugs (foreign substances) is in direct opposition to physiological law, and has no scientific foundation whatever.

From the countless remedies of the pharmacopceia we can select substances that if administered to a healthy person will produce almost any known form of disease thus: brandy, cayenne pepper and quinine, will induce inflammatory fever; scammony and ipecac will cause cholera morbus; nitre, calomel and opium, will provoke typhoid or typhus fever; digitalis will cause Asiatic, or spasmodic cholera; cod liver oil and sulphur promote scurvy, and all the cathartic family inevitably cause diarrhcea, the disease in each case being nothing more than the effort of Nature to get rid of these troublesome intruders.

Drugs do not, as their advocates claim, select their special organ with a view of acting upon it, but are acted upon by that particular organ for the purpose of ridding the system of the drug.

It follows, therefore, as a perfectly legitimate and logical deduction, that, if the system of administering drugs is founded upon a wrong conception of their relation to the human organism, then any theoretical "law of cure" predicated upon drug action must necessarily be equally fallacious and untrustworthy.

As stated before, the simple fact is, that there is no law of cure, only a condition and that condition--obedience, by which is meant a course of treatment in harmony with Nature.

The older physicians grow the more they rely upon the vis medicatrix naturae, which is, after all, the only remedial force, and one totally beyond their control. The physician can no more perform cures than the farmer can make his crops grow. In each case, all that can be done is to employ all the methods that cumulative wisdom can suggest to make the conditions as favorable as possible, and leave the rest to Mother Nature, who is not in the habit of making mistakes, and whose unerring methods would cure ninety per cent. of all diseased conditions, if her beneficent intentions were not frustrated by well-meant, but nevertheless pernicious, drug interference.

PART II.

THE TRUE CAUSE OF DISEASE.

At this point the reader will doubtless be tempered to exclaim: "Well, you have demonstrated to your own satisfaction that the medical profession entertains erroneous opinions as to the true nature of disease, and also that drugs are absolutely useless--nay, injurious--in such conditions: but is this all? Having destroyed our trust in drugs, what have you to offer in their stead?"

To which perfectly natural query, I gladly reply, I have a system of treatment to propound, a system that has triumphantly stood the test of years, a system that must commend itself to every intelligent reader, because it is strictly in accordance with natural law.

But before I proceed to explain it, I desire to announce my own theory respecting disease--a theory essentially radical in its character, and of which I am the originator, and that is:

THERE IS ONLY ONE CAUSE OF DISEASE.

This may sound strange, for the majority of people imagine that there is a different and specific cause for every ailment, and physicians generally do not combat the opinion. But as a matter of fact, there is only one disease, although its manifestations are various, and there is only one cause for it, and that is the retention of waste matters in the system. These substances may be in the gaseous, liquid or solid form, but they are foreign bodies, inimical to the welfare of the organism, and their presence must result in derangement of bodily function.

The great need of the present day is adequate instruction in physiology and hygiene, that humanity may not only know how to secure the restoration of health, when lost, but by attention to physiological and sanitary laws may retain good health indefinitely. The body is the theatre of constant change. The process of tearing down and building up proceed without intermission during life. If construction exceeds destruction, the result is health; but just as surely as destruction exceeds repair, disease is the result. But during every moment of life waste is being formed by the destruction of tissue, and this effete material must be promptly removed if the individual would enjoy health. Nature has provided adequate means for the removal of these substances which are valueless to the economy, the retention of which obstructs and irritates the complex mechanism of the system, the principal avenues for its expulsion being the lungs, the skin and the intestinal canal. The latter is infinitely more important than the others, since by it the waste products of digestion are expelled. If it fails to promptly fulfil its office, every vital function is interfered with; and in addition the fluid portion of the semi-liquid waste is re-absorbed directly into the circulation, redepositing in the very fountain of life, matter which the system has thrown off as worthless.

Should the system be exposed to a chill, while in this condition, a congestion of the surface excretory vessels takes place; and practically the whole work of elimination is thrown upon the already hard-worked kidneys, frequently resulting in uraemic poisoning and death.

The presence of a grain of sand in a watch will retard its movements, if not arrest them altogether. What, then, must be the result of an accumulation of impurities in the physical system? The finely adjusted balance that is capable of weighing the thousandth part of a grain, is carefully protected under a glass cover, for even impalpable dust would clog its movements. Reflect, then, upon the amount of friction that must be perpetually going on in the human organism owing to the retention of effete matter! And since not even the most cunning product of man's handiwork can compare with the intricate mechanism of the body, the importance of eliminating the waste becomes manifest. Here, in a nutshell, lies the secret of disease.

Let us now consider how the retention of waste affects the system--how the deleterious effects are produced. There are three factors at work in this process, mechanical, gaseous and absorptive, the last named being infinitely the most pernicious. We will first consider the mechanical.

Nature has beautifully apportioned the space in the abdominal cavity, each part of the viscera having ample room for the performance of its special function, but any abnormal increase in size of any part of the contents of the cavity must necessarily create disturbance. Now, when the food leaves the stomach, where it has been churned into a pulpaceous mass, it passes into the duodenum or second stomach, where it receives an augmentation of liquid material from the liver and pancreas; consequently, when it reaches the small intestine, where absorption takes place, it is in a well diluted condition. During its passage through the small intestine, the nutrient portion of the ingesta is abstracted from it by the villi (small hair-like processes) with which the small intestine is thickly studded, so that at the end of its journey of about twenty-two feet (if digestion is normal) all that is of value to the organism has been appropriated--the remainder being refuse. This waste product passes into the colon, or large intestine, and should be promptly expelled. If prompt expulsion does not take place, this is what happens: The fluid portion of this semi- liquid waste is re-absorbed through the walls of the colon directly into the circulation, a percentage of the solids being deposited on the walls of the intestine. This process of accretion goes on from day to day, week to week, month to month, until it not infrequently happens that the colon becomes distended to several times its natural size. Instances are on record, where these abnormal accumulations of faecal matter in the colon have been mistaken for enlargement of the liver, and even pregnancy. A surgeon in London has a preparation of the colon measuring some twenty inches in circumference, containing three gallons of faecal matter, and even larger accumulations have been reported. The foregoing instances are, of course, exceptional ones, but it is safe to assert that seventy per cent. of the colons of the human family (living under civilized conditions) are impacted, and some of them terribly so. It is impossible to estimate the amount of evil caused by an engorged colon monopolizing two or three times its allotted space in the abdominal cavity, crowding and hampering the other organs in their work.

But the effects of direct mechanical pressure are not the only ones. The accumulations in the colon necessarily arrest the free passage of the product of the small intestine, and that, in turn, causes undue retention of food in the stomach, with consequent fermentation; while the irritation, due to pressure on the nerve terminals by the distension, and by the encrusted matter adhering to the intestinal wall, is simply incalculable.

The effects of gaseous accumulations in the alimentary canal are not thoroughly understood at present--that is--the pathological effects. The more direct effects, as manifested in abdominal distension, and the terrible distress that frequently follows eating, are unfortunately, but too well known. The reader does not need to be told that during the decomposition of organic substances, gases are evolved, and no matter where the process goes on, the results are always the same. Owing to the causes previously mentioned, the intestinal canal usually offers special facilities for the production of gases, owing to the retention of partially digested food, in a medium highly favorable to fermentation. A moderate amount of sulphuretted hydrogen, and also carburetted hydrogen is always present in the colon, normally, to preserve moderate distention of the walls, while the gases usually found in the stomach and small intestine, are oxygen, hydrogen, nitrogen and carbonic acid. What functional disturbances may arise from the presence of these gaseous substances in excess in the system is, at present, largely a matter of conjecture, but it is known that a stream of carbonic acid gas, or hydrogen continuously directed against a muscle will cause paralysis of that structure. The expansive force of gases is too well known to need comment, and the force with which they will at times distend the abdominal wall points irresistibly to the conclusion that such an amount of force exerted against vital organs cannot be otherwise than productive of serious harm. It is not at all improbable that many cases of hernia and uterine displacement may be due to this hitherto unsuspected cause. That they penetrate the neighboring tissues is an established fact, and it is quite conceivable that their action upon the nervous system though the medium of the circulation may lie at the root of many of the cases of neurasthenia that are now so prevalent.

But the auto-infection that results from the absorption of the liquid waste into the blood supply is by far the most serious feature. The blood is the life. From it the system obtains all the material for the formation of fresh tissue, and it is a practical impossibility for good, healthy structures to be built up from a tainted blood current. Why is it that the vegetation on the banks of a stream, on which a manufacturing town is located, is invariably stunted and withered? Because the water that should nourish it is polluted by the refuse poured into it, and no amount of deodorants or disinfectants will prove of any avail to restore the devitalized vegetation, but will rather aggravate the trouble. But cut off the source of pollution, and in an incredibly short space of time the vegetation will take on a new 1ease of life.

This liquid refuse in the colon is composed of substances for which the system has no further use--it has rejected them; consequently they are foreign bodies, and as such, are the equivalent of poisons. The colon, in this condition, is a perfect hot-bed for the breeding of all kinds of poisonous germs, and the action of cathartics aggravates the condition by filling the pouched portions of the colon with a foul liquid which facilitates the absorption of the ptomaines and leucomaines through the mucous coat of the intestine. It is known now, that as much as three-fourths of this foul putrid substance may be absorbed, carrying into the system poisonous germs and excrementitious matter. Dr. Murchison states, "that a circulation is constantly taking place between the fluid contents of the bowel and the blood, the existence of which, till within the last few years, was quite unknown, and which even now is too little heeded." And Dr. Parker says, "It is now known, that in varying degrees there is a constant transit of fluid from the blood into the alimentary canal, and as rapid absorption." It is also stated on reliable authority, "that every portion of the blood may, and possibly does, pass several times into the alimentary canal in twenty-four hours." Prof. I. I. Metchinkoff recently stated in a lecture at Paris: "Particularly injurious are the microbes of the large intestines. Thence, they penetrate into the blood and impair it alike by their presence and the products they yield--ptomaines, alkaloids, etc. The auto intoxication of the organism and poisoning through microbes is an established fact."

Having shown that the average colon is a fertile breeding ground for all kinds of poisonous germs, and that they are conveyed into the circulation by the interchange of fluids in that organ, it may be interesting to explain how these germs are conveyed to, and deposited in the various organs of the body.

We have in our bodies a system of canals called arteries and veins, having their head at the heart, which is the main pump that keeps the blood in motion. The arterial circulation consists of those channels which convey the blood--supposed pure blood--away from the heart to the different parts of the body, loaded with the life-giving principle of sustenance, invigoration and heat, while the veins or venous circulation conveys to the heart and lungs the impure blood, loaded many times with disease-breeding germs.

Now, in the blood, as it courses through our bodies, are myriads of little vessels called corpuscles; these are what give the blood a red color. There are also a smaller number of white corpuscles, that are known as phagocytes, whose mission is to destroy micro-organisms that are prejudicial to life. In order that you may know their use, I, for convenience sake and to make my meaning better understood, will call them little war vessels, loaded with soldiers, and the soldiers have in their vessels a furnace whose fire never goes out. These vessels and their little warriors are continually sailing through our bodies, hunting for germs of disease, that they catch and throw into their furnace and burn them up. Now, suppose we take a violent cold, thus closing the pores of the skin, and that at the same time the colon is engorged, two of the most important outlets for the filth and decayed matter of our bodies are closed up--for the life of our bodies is one continual process of building anew and tearing down; these two most important sewers are now closed. These little vessels now have their hands full, catching disease-bearing germs that nature cannot throw out through the colon or pores of the skin--both being closed--and we call this condition of things fever. The white corpuscle has but two dumping places now, the lungs or kidneys. Suppose that in the colon is the tubercular ulcer, breeding the bacillus of consumption, and they are absorbed into the circulation. Ordinarily the white corpuscles would be able to destroy them, but now they are so overworked that the tubercular germ lands in the lung tissue alive and well, ready to commence his work of destruction and death. The person developes a hacking cough, and finally goes to the doctor, and he, if he knows his business, probably finds tuberculosis well established. Typhoid fever has its nursery solely in the colon, and gets possession of the citadel of life in the same way as any other germ or contagious disease. What a terrible battle there must be going on in us between our life-preservers and the germs of disease.

Is it any wonder that people die of premature old age, of apoplexy, paralysis, dropsy, consumption, and the thousand and one maladies that scourge humanity? And is it not unreasonable to pour a few grains of diluted drugs into the stomach to purify the blood--even granting for the sake of argument that such a purpose could be accomplished by that means--when occupying nearly one-half of the abdominal cavity is an engorged intestine reeking with filth so foul that carrion is as the odor of roses compared to it, and which is being steadily absorbed into the circulation? If a man were to act as foolishly as that in his business, his friends would quickly petition the courts to appoint a guardian for him.

It may be asked, why has not this discovery been made before? In the first place, the colon has had but scant attention paid to it in the dissecting room, until of late years the appendicitis craze has awakened some interest in it. Its importance was not realized--the circulatory and nervous systems receiving the lion's share of attention. In the second place, in holding post-mortems the organ was avoided, cut off, if in the way, and thrown into the slop bucket. It was known to be always full, but no one ever asked whether or not it was natural in its fullness of faecal matter, and as a result, probably the profession knows the least about this important organ, of any in the human body. Strange, is it not, that among the seven thousand physicians ground out and polished in the mills of wisdom each year, that there was not one who had originality enough to ask the question, Is it natural that this scent bag of filth should always be so full of putrid matter that we cannot abide one moment with it? And, inasmuch as it is so, is it not a great detriment at least to our health to carry this mass of filth around with us, from day to day, from week to week, and from year to year--absorbing its poison back into the circulation? Strange that these questions did not present themselves to some one of the enterprising youths of our original young America.

The muscular fibres of the intestines are circular and longitudinal. In the large intestine the longitudinal fibres are shorter than the tube itself, which length permits the formation of loculi (cavities). These become the seat of faecal accumulations, only too often unnoticed by the physician. It is undoubtedly a fact that the loculi of the colon contain small faecal accumulations extending over weeks, months, or even years. Their presence produces symptoms varying all the way from a little catarrhal irritation up to the most diverse, and in some instances serious, reflex disturbances. When the loculi only are filled, the main channel of the colon is undisturbed. The most common parts of the colon to become enlarged are the sigmoid flexure and the caecum (see diagram in beginning of book), but accumulations may occur in any part of the colon. The ascending colon is much more often filled in life than the books would lead us to believe; indeed, it may be said that chronic accumulations are oftener to be found in the ascending than in the descending colon, which is also contrary to the assertions of the authors. This is due partly to the fact that the contents of the colon have to rise in opposition to gravity, and partly to the semi-paralyzed condition of the muscular coat of the colon through inactivity. When the accumulations are large, the increased weight of the colon tends to displace it; and if in the transverse colon, that portion may be depressed, even into the pelvis.

The mass may be so enormous as to press upon any organ located in the abdomen, interfering with its functions; thus we may have pressure on the liver that arrests the flow of bile; or, upon the urinary organs, crippling their functions.

Of course, such excessive accumulations occur only exceptionally, and it is not to these that attention is particularly drawn, because when they are so excessive, any physician can detect them by palpation (touch).

It is to the minor accumulations particularly, that I wish to draw attention--the accumulations that we see in the majority of patients who visit our offices. Such patients assure us that the bowels move daily, but the color of their complexions, and the condition of their tongues, are enough to assure us that they are the victims of costiveness.

Daily movements of the bowels are no sign that the colon is not impacted; in fact, the worst cases of costiveness that we ever see are those in which daily movements of the bowels occur. The diagnosis of faecal accumulations is facilitated by inquiring as to the color of the daily discharges. A black or a very dark green color almost always indicates the faeces are ancient.

Prompt discharge of food refuse is indicated by more or less yellow color. It would be interesting to inquire why fresh faces are yellow and ancient faeces are dark.

Such patients have digestive fermentations to torment them, resulting in flatulent distension which encroaches on the cavity of the chest, which in excessive cases may cause short and rapid breathing, irregular heart action, disturbed circulation in the brain, with vertigo and headache. An over-distended caecum, or sigmoid flexure, from pressure, may produce dropsy, numbness or cramps in the right or left lower extremity.

The reports of the Post-mortem examination of the colons of hundreds of subjects reveals a series of horrors more weird and ghastly than were ever penned by Eugene Sue, or Emile Zola. The mind shrinks in dismay at the appalling revelations, and shudders at the possibly of the "human form divine" becoming such a peripatetic charnel house.

Is it any wonder that the average human system, being thus saturated with impurities, should succumb to the first exciting cause? Is it not, in fact, a greater marvel that the rate of mortality is not even higher than at present?

My object in publishing this book is to point out the true cause of disease, together with the means for its prevention and cure, and that, too, by a simple and inexpensive method of hygienic treatment, which has proved eminently successful in tens of thousands of cases, which is perfectly harmless and natural in its action, and absolutely free from even the suspicion of a drug.

PART III.

RATIONAL HYGIENIC TREATMENT.

Having striven to explain in an intelligible manner the true nature and cause of disease, and to point out the inadequacy of the drug system of treatment to combat pathological conditions successfully (not from any lack of intention on the part of the drug practitioners: but from the unreliability of their methods), I shall now proceed to lay before you the system of treatment which it is proposed to substitute in its stead, and I unhesitatingly affirm that it will be found so simple, so inexpensive and so obviously based on common sense and true hygienic principles, that the thoughtful reader cannot fail to give it his unqualified endorsement, and will be lost in wonder that any one should fail to adopt it, when made acquainted with its simplicity and its marvellous results.

In an old comedy, which used to delight our fore-fathers, the hero, Felix O'Callaghan, defines the practice of medicine as "the art of amusing the patient while Nature performs the cure." In that sentence, the dramatist (unwittingly perhaps) embodied a great truth. Nature, and Nature only, can effect a cure. Fresh air, sunlight, pure water, diet and exercise are the great curative agents provided by Nature, and all that the physician can do, no matter to what school be belongs, is to remove as far as possible all existing impediments, and to see that the hygienic conditions are made as favorable as possible. For the rest, Nature, the marvellous builder, will, in her own mysterious way, build up fresh tissue, and, slowly but surely, repair the ravages made by disease. No one would dare to say that the farmer made the corn grow. He does all that the science of agriculture tells him is needful to furnish proper conditions for growth, but there he must stop--the rest must be left to Nature. Then, since disease is a wasting of tissue, and recovery a building up, it is a palpable absurdity to credit a physician with a cure. All that he can do is to cooperate with Nature, by seeing that none of her laws are violated, and insisting that nothing whatever shall obstruct her beneficent functions.

Whether for the preservation of health, or the treatment of disease, when present, the chief thing is to cleanse the colon. It is useless to attempt to get rid of the effects while the cause is present.

If the principal drain in a dwelling becomes choked, what is the consequence?

The noxious and pestilent gases generated by the accumulated filth having no outlet, are forced back into the building, poisoning the atmosphere, and breeding contagion among the inhabitants. Deodorizing and disinfecting will simply be a waste of time and material, until the drain is cleared. The colon is the main drain of the human body, and if it be necessary, for sanitary reasons, to keep the house drains clean, how vitally important is it to keep the main outlet of the physical system free from obstructions.

Or, to use another homely illustration, when your coal stove has been run continuously for a long time, as a natural result it becomes clogged with cinders and ashes, causing the fire to burn badly. You encourage it with fresh fuel, rake it and shake it but without avail--the accumulations of debris are too great. You remove a portion, but its place is taken by more substance from above. At length you resort to the measure you should have employed at first--you "dump the grate" and start a fresh fire. The moral is obvious: dump the grate of the human system--in other words, empty the colon.

It has been previously shown that an impacted colon is neither more nor less than a prolific hot-bed for the wholesale breeding of disease germs--microbes--those infinitesimal organisms which science has demonstrated to be the cause of many phases of disease, or rather, the toxins (poisons) they produce, cause disease. Of course, there are harmless micro-organisms as well as hurtful ones; in fact, a large proportion of them are beneficial rather than otherwise; but some of them (notably the tubercle bacillus) are so intimately associated with disease that it is next to impossible to doubt their responsibility.

The sphere of the microbe is absolutely without limit. He is equally at ease in the air, the earth, and the water. He makes himself at home in our beverages and our foods. Our mouths furnish desirable lurking places for him, our hair, and finger-nails are favorite posts of vantage; while he delights to disport himself in our blood. He is the active agent of decay, and the prime cause of disease. He is the most selfish of parasites. The world for a long time disregarded him, but now acknowledges him as one of the mightiest of conquerers; for while other devastators have slain thousands, millions have fallen beneath his insidious attacks. He is a foe to be dreaded, for he is forever lying in ambush for fresh victims.

Microbes breed in fermentation, consequently, every particle of undigested food remaining in the stomach or intestines becomes an ideal nursery for their propagation. It has been demonstrated that food that has been subjected to the action of the gastric juice decomposes far more rapidly than that which has not--hence, with imperfect digestion, fermentation quickly takes place. If microbes are now introduced into the system, either by contact with sick persons, inhaling impure air in crowded public buildings, or breathing in the dust on ill-kept streets, there is danger ahead; for if the recipient is not in a sound, physical condition, the microbes (finding congenial lodgment), multiply with the most marvellous rapidity, permeating every portion of the tissue--causing, in fact, DECOMPOSITION WHILE STILL ALIVE.

Every particle of animal or vegetable matter, even if only a single grain in weight, by exposure to the air, putrefies, breeds, and attracts to itself thousands of microbes, and becomes a center of infection. Thus, in a piece of street dirt containing organic matter, we may find upon examination, the germs of typhoid fever, diphtheria, scarlet fever, or consumption. When this piece of dirt is dried by the sun and pulverized by horses' hoofs, the particles of dirt are caught up by the wind, and sent whirling through the air, to be drawn into the lungs by those within reach, Of course, every one who breathes in the microbes of some particular disease does not catch it, or we should soon all be dead, but those who have not the resisting power of sound bodies to kill these germs, before they have time to set up their peculiar inflammation, are apt to realize the evil effects, a week, a month, or even a year afterwards.

It is evident then that to cure disease we must get rid of all fermentation in the system, and thus prevent the further breeding of microbes and to prevent disease we must get the system into such a sound, healthy condition that disease germs cannot obtain a lodgment in it.

Now, this can only be accomplished by thoroughly cleansing the colon, and keeping it absolutely clean, thus preventing further contamination of the blood current--the fountain of life.

The intelligent reader, recognizing the absolute correctness of the foregoing proposition, will naturally ask, "Can such a thing be accomplished, and how?" We beg to assure the reader, most emphatically, that it can, but not by the means usually employed. It is perfectly plain that the cleansing process cannot be effected by cathartics, for at the best, they only afford temporary relief (witness the growth of the cathartic habit), while on an impacted mass such as is commonly present in the colon, the influence they can exert is practically nil. The common experience of those afflicted with constipation is, that they commence with a laxative, gradually increasing the quantity and frequency of the dose until it fails to act at all. Then they resort to a cathartic, with a similar experience, when it is exchanged for a more powerful one, and then for another still more powerful, until at last, it becomes impossible to move the bowels without a powerful dose.

That this is no overdrawn picture many of my readers will bear witness, and my brother practitioners can amply corroborate the statement, for they fully recognize the vital importance of removing the waste from the system. The pity of it is that they still persist in employing such a crude and ineffective method.

Do any of my readers know how a cathartic acts?

It is popularly supposed that the drug passes from the stomach into the small intestines, rendering their contents more liquid; then passes into the colon, producing the same effect upon its more solid contents, thus causing an evacuation. Many people have no conception, whatever, of the modus operandi of a purgative drug, simply believing that it acts in a certain mysterious manner, but the above described process is generally believed to be the correct one by those who have thought upon the matter, but lack physiological knowledge. It is a huge mistake.

Any purgative drug, whether aperient, laxative or cathartic, is dissolved in the stomach by the action of the gastric juice--in fact, goes through the same digestive process as the food that is eaten, that is, it passes into the small intestines and is there absorbed into the circulation.

By its irritation of the nerves, the secretory and excretory processes of the system are stimulated into abnormal action, and an extra quantity of fluid is poured into the colon to dissolve the accumulated mass; which is about as scientific a proceeding as pouring a quart of water into a washbowl on the upper floor of a dwelling to clear away an obstruction in the main drain of the building. And, again, as previously stated, the action of laxatives and cathartics, especially the variety known as hydrogo-cathartics (watery), fill the ano-rectal cavity and the loculi, or folds of the colon, with a foul watery solution that is a perpetual source of irritation to the sensitive mucous surface, hastening and intensifying the process of auto-infection by absorption, that is constantly going on.

And what about the enormous drain upon the vital forces? Who is not familiar with the feeling of exhaustion when the reaction sets in after the employment of such methods of relief? How can it be otherwise? These stimulants to defecation are like the applications of the whip to the jaded horse-they excite the system to make a supreme effort in the required direction, but the reaction is disastrous in the extreme. With the repeated demands upon the delicate nervous system incidental to constant catharsis is it any wonder that we are so constantly confronted with cases of nervous collapse? The wonder would be if it were otherwise.

Nor are these the only objections to be urged against purgative medication. Its effects upon the digestive functions is, in the highest degree, destructive. It would be next to impossible to find an individual addicted to the use of cathartics whose digestion was not, practically, a wreck. It is true, that a large part of the digestive disturbance in such cases is due to the obstructed condition of the colon, and the consequent undue retention of food in the stomach, until fermentation sets in; but no inconsiderable share of the trouble is due to the action of the drugs, by repeated over- stimulation of the nervous system, and perpetual irritation of the delicate absorbent vessels.

Viewed from whatever standpoint we may choose, the employment of drugs to relieve an overcharged colon is both unsatisfactory and unscientific.

And yet there is a simple and effective method of dealing with this trouble; of removing the accumulations, no matter how large they may be; of thoroughly cleansing and purifying that important organ, the colon, without the least demand upon the vital forces, and that is by

WASHING IT OUT.

In plain English, the preservation and restoration of health depends entirely upon cleanliness, especially internal cleanliness, and to attain that condition which we are told is next to godliness, there is nothing equal to water--especially "hot water, which is the great scavenger of nature."

Strange, that such an obviously common-sense proceeding should not be universal, is it not? I do not claim to be the discoverer of this method of internal purification, for it is in reality of ancient origin, as we have it on good authority that it was practised by the ancient Egyptians, who, it is believed, acquired their knowledge from observing a bird called the Ibis, a species of Egyptian snipe. The food of this bird, gathered on the banks of the Nile, was of a very constipating character, and it was observed, by the earliest naturalists, to suck up the water of the river and using its long bill for a syringe, inject it into its anus, thus relieving itself. Pliny says this habit of the Ibis first suggested the use of clysters to the ancient Egyptian doctors, known to be the first medical practitioners of any nation, not excepting the Chinese. [See Naturalis Historia, Lib. VIII., Dap. 41, Hague 1518.

Another writer, viz., Christianus Langius, says, that this bird when attacked with constipation at some distance from the river, and not able to fly from weakness, would be seen to crawl to the water's edge with drooping wings and there take its rectal treatment, when in a few minutes it would fly away in full vigor of regained strength.

Nor do I even claim to have rediscovered this system of treatment, although it is a common practice in these days to revamp old theories and discoveries, and try to foist them upon the public as entirely new propositions. The credit for the resuscitation of this ancient remedial practice belongs, without doubt, to Dr. A. Wilford Hall, of New York, who practiced the treatment on himself for forty years before giving its principles to the public, thereby fully proving its merits.

The following experience from the pen of Dr. H. T. Turner, of Washington, affords incontestable proof of the allegation made, that the colon is the seat of disease, and his testimony should be read with extreme care. It is no fanciful, theoretical statement, but the ghastly revelation of an appalling reality. While reading his statement, the reader will do well to refer to the engraving, representing the digestive apparatus, at the commencement of this book, as it will greatly facilitate his comprehension of the matter.

"In 1880 I lost a patient with inflammation of the bowels, and requested of the friends the privilege of holding a post-mortem examination, as I was satisfied that there was some foreign substance in or near the Ileo-coecal valve, or in that apparently useless appendage, the Appendicula Vermiformis. (See explanation of engraving.)

"The autopsy developed a quantity of grape seed and popcorn, filling the lower enlarged pouch of the colon and the opening into the Appendicula Vermiformis. This, from the mortified and blackened condition of the colon alone, indicated that my diagnosis was correct. I opened the colon throughout its entire length of five feet, and found it filled with faecal matter encrusted on its walls and into the folds of the colon, in many places dry and hard as slate, and so completely obstructing the passage of the bowels as to throw him into violent colic (as his friends stated), sometimes as often as twice a month, for years, and that powerful doses of physic was his only relief; that all the doctors had agreed that it was bilious colic. I observed that this crusted matter was evidently of long standing, the result of years of accumulation, and although the remote cause, not the immediate cause of his death. The sigmoid-flexure (see engraving), or bend in the colon on the left side, was especially full, and distended to double its natural size, filling the gut uniformly, with a small hole the size of one's little finger through the center, through which the recent faecal matter passed. In the lower part of the sigmoid-flexure, just before descending to form the rectum, and in the left hand upper corner of the colon as it turns toward the right, were pockets eaten out of the hardened faecal matter, in which were eggs of worms and quite a quantity of maggots, which had eaten into the sensitive mucous membrane, causing serious inflammation of the colon and its adjacent parts, and as recent investigation has established as a fact, were the cause of his hemorrhoids, or piles, which I learned were of years' standing. The whole length of the colon was in a state of chronic inflammation; still this man considered himself well and healthy until the unfortunate eating of the grape seed and popcorn, and had no trouble in getting his life insured in one of the best companies in America.

"I have been thus explicit in this description, from the fact that recent investigation has developed the fact that in the discovery described above, I had found but a prototype of at least seven-tenths of the human family in civilized life--the real cause of all diseases of the human body, excepting the grape seed and popcorn. That I had found the fountain of premature old age and death, for, as surprising as it may seem, out of 284 cases of autopsies held of late on the colon (they representing in their death nearly all the diseases known to our climate), but twenty-eight colons were found to be free from hardened, adhered matter, and in their normal healthy state, and that the 256 were all more or less as described above, except, perhaps, the grape seeds and popcorn. In many of them the colon was distended to double its natural size throughout its whole length, with a small hole through the center, and as far as could be learned, these last cases spoken of had regular evacuations of the bowels each day. Many of the colons contained large maggots from four to six inches long, and pockets of eggs and maggots, while blood and pus were frequently present."

The question is often asked, and naturally so, why this unnatural accumulation is in the colon? The horse and ox promptly obey the call of nature; they know no time or place, and are blessed with clean colons. So are the natives of Africa. But the demands of civilized life insist upon a time and place. Business, etiquette, opportunity, and a thousand and one excuses stand continually in the way, and nature's call is put off to a more convenient time and place.

How many people are not presentable to themselves or friends, owing to the putrid smell of their bodies, so that in polite society strong colognes and other perfumes are used. Show me a woman who girts her waist with corsets or any tight clothing, and I will warrant you that the smell from her body will be sickening in the extreme. The special reason for this is, that the lacing comes immediately where the transverse colon crosses her body. Now, if the sigmoid-flexure becomes loaded, because of its folding upon itself, how much more will the transverse colon become clogged if unnaturally folded upon itself by compression from each side folding it, as demonstrated in some instances, almost double the whole length, into two extra elbows, where it, if natural; is straight (see engraving on next page). Many reasons have been given by physiologists and humanitarians, why it is injurious for the lady to lace, but this reason outweighs them all. Wear the clothing loose, clean out the colon and heal it up, and you will smell sweet, and life will be a continual blessing; for if the main sewer in the body is closed or clogged, nature has but three other outlets: the capillaries or pores of the skin, the lungs in exhalation, or the kidneys. If the colon is clogged, the penned-up acid permeations of the stomach and duodenum will have to seek other outlets, which is indicated by the putrid smell of the body and a foul breath with finally dyspepsia, and what is usually termed biliousness, torpid liver, etc.

The condition of the colon (the physiological sewer) in the average adult having been demonstrated, does it need any argument to convince the intelligent thinker that the most rational and practical manner of dealing with this hot-bed of filth and breeding place of disease, is to wash it out?

With me, it has passed beyond the theoretical stage, for I have in my office fully 15,000 grateful letters from patients who have used this process, under my direction, with the most astounding results; scarcely a disease known to humanity, but has been relieved, and in ninety-five per cent. of cases, cures effected; while tens of thousands of gratifying messages have reached me from time to time; nor is the testimony in its favor confined to the laity, for hundreds of physicians (including some of the most prominent authorities) testify to the wonderfully beneficial results achieved by its use.

We now come to the most important feature of the subject--the means for putting it into practice, for it will readily be admitted that such an admirable and common-sense method of treatment should have the most perfect means procurable for its application, but until the present time the available means have remained crude and undeveloped. This, however, is scarcely to be wondered at. It is the history of all important discoveries.

Those great natural forces, steam and electricity, although their value was recognized, yet required the aid of inventive genius to develop their possibilities; in fact, it has required three-fourths of a century to bring the locomotive to its present state of perfection, while the potentialities of electricity are as yet only surmised. This being so in matters that offer a rich pecuniary harvest to the inventor, it is little matter for surprise that improvement in a means of combating disease should progress slowly. In the first place, it was a new departure, unheralded to the world, and frowned upon by the members of the orthodox medical schools; consequently there was no tempting bait of a handsome profit to encourage the inventor, and until lately the indifference to matters pertaining to health was proverbial.

When Dr. Hall commenced his famous experimentation upon himself, the only appliance available for the purpose was the old-fashioned bulb syringe, which is simply a flexible rubber tube with an egg-shaped receptacle in the center. One end of the tube is inserted in the rectum, while the other end is immersed in a vessel of water, the injection of the fluid being accomplished by alternately compressing and relaxing the bulbous portion. It is needless to say that the process of "flushing the colon" copiously, the only effectual way, was a tedious, inconvenient and imperfect matter with such a crude appliance. After the lapse of a great number of years the "gravity" or "fountain" syringe was invented, which consisted of a rubber bag with a long flexible tube attached to its lower end. The bag was suspended from a nail or hook several feet above the individual, the water being forced into the body by gravity, the pressure being increased or diminished by raising or lowering the bag. This was a distinct advance upon the bulb syringe, but it still left a great deal to be desired. In the first place, they are both exceedingly tedious, a serious objection in the case of weakly or elderly people; secondly, both methods necessitate the uncovering of the lower portion of the body, which is decidedly unpleasant; and, most serious of all, it is impossible to prevent the admission of air into the intestine, and that is a fruitful source of pain and discomfort. It should, however, be borne in mind that both of these appliances were devised for an entirely different class of operation (namely, vaginal douching), and were only used for intestinal treatment because there was nothing better at hand.

Another method, sometimes employed by progressive physicians, consists in using, in connection with the fountain syringe, a tube from eighteen to twenty-four inches in length, made of a firm but flexible variety of rubber. This was introduced (its entire length) into the body, the theory being that it was necessary to get behind the impacted mass and force it out ahead of the water, which was theoretically correct, but in practice found sadly wanting. In the first place, the opening in the eye of the tube became clogged with the faecal matter, and, secondly, with the double tube employed for the return flow, the opening was too small to allow of the passage of solid substances. The introduction of the catheter is a process requiring considerable skill, and a perfect acquaintance with the anatomy of the parts, so that personal use of it is practically impossible, or, at least, attended with considerable danger. An examination of the diagram of the digestive apparatus at the beginning of the book will enable the reader to understand the difficulties attending its introduction, since it has to pass the sigmoid flexure (No. 12), and the splenic flexure--that angle of the colon where the transverse portion turns to descend. With such a tortuous road to travel, the risk of injury to the sensitive mucous membrane is excessive--hence this instrument should never be used by the patient upon himself.

The author, however, felt that there must be an easier and more effective method of irrigating that important organ--the colon--and one unattended with any risk, and determined, if possible, to devise some better way. After much patient and tireless experimenting he invented and perfected the "J. B. L. Cascade," a mechanical appliance which completely rids the process of all its objectionable features, and enables young and old, weak and strong, to use the treatment without the possibility of danger. It achieves the desired result far more effectively than any other known apparatus, with the least possible inconvenience to the patient, and yet so gently and easily that the operation, so far from being distressing or disagreeable, becomes a positive gratification.

The letters J. B. L. are the initials of the words Joy, Beauty, Life, which aptly indicate its purpose and effects, for we confidently claim that its use will infallibly confer these three great blessings, it being the one safe and sanative method of regaining and preserving health. Without health there is no joy in life, and perfect beauty cannot possibly exist, while with health life becomes indeed worth living.

One of the gravest objections to all the hitherto existing appliances is the construction of the nozzle, or tube, that is inserted in the body, and through which the water is conveyed. These are all (without exception) made with an aperature in the end, or extreme tip, the consequence being that a small jet of water is continuously directed upon one spot in the delicate and sensitive mucous membrane. With water at the necessary temperature this is a source of grave danger, and likely to result in serious injury, by causing a separation of the various layers of which the membrane is composed. When this separation occurs little slits occur in the rectal lining, in which faecal matter lodges, ultimately forming what are known as pockets, causing, first, irritation, then inflammation, and, finally, results in "proctitis"-- chronic inflammation of the intestinal canal. The best authorities agree in condemning the direct jet, while rectal specialists regard it as one of their chief aids to income.

With these facts in view, the construction of my "injection point," or entering tube, engaged the special attention, finally, with the result that a most successful means of overcoming this dangerous objection has been provided. Instead of the opening in the end, the tip is made absolutely solid, so that the impact of the entering water is not felt at all, while it is provided with six rows of perforations on the sides, through which the water is evenly diffused over the walls of the rectum, which is a most desirable thing in cases of hemorrhoids or rectal inflammations. It is also so constructed that the natural constriction of the sphincter muscles holds it firmly in position in the rectum, and while affording the water free passage into the colon, it prevents the escape of the fluid externally, thus rendering soiled garments impossible.

But the simplicity of the operation is one of its chief advantages, for the patient sits upon the appliance in ease and comfort while receiving the cleansing stream, and by following the directions the time occupied in the operation need not exceed fifteen minutes, or about one-fourth of the time required by other methods--an unmistakably valuable saving of time and strain to busy or weakly people. The faucet is considered by experts as a most valuable feature, on account of the "dome" portion, which accurately fits the natural arch formed by the limbs when the body is in the seated position.

Many people are accustomed to use the bulb and fountain syringes in a reclining position and some physicians recommend the patient to kneel in the bath tub, with the body bent well forward: an irksome, disagreeable position and quite unnecessary. The theory is, that the water will flow into the body by gravitation, but they overlook the fact that the ascending and descending portions of the colon, being parallel in the body, the water, while flowing readily into the descending portions, would have to flow uphill in the ascending portions and by the time it reached there, the force would be exhausted. The weight of the body furnishes greater force, which is proportioned to the size and bulk of the patient, but is not perceptible to him, on account of the solid construction of the tip of the "injection point," while the steady, uniform pressure exerted serves to distend the walls of the colon and thus liberate adherent matter. By far the great majority of people, however, use these crude appliances while seated over a vessel, which is decidedly injurious. By reference to the diagram of the digestive organs it will be seen that the "descending colon," that portion which terminates in the rectum, is larger than either of the other divisions of that organ. In fact, its capacity (in the average adult) is about three pints, equivalent to three pounds. Now this weight, in a flexible organ like the colon, must cause a sagging down, exerting a serious strain upon its attachments to the abdominal wall, and by its pressure upon the sphincters will induce prolapse of the rectum. That is one reason why so many people find it almost impossible to receive enough water to make the treatment successful. When a physician, or trained nurse, is administering a high enema, it is a common practice to hold a folded towel against the rectum, to guard against this pressure and its possible results. The "dome" portion of the faucet (previously referred to) affords the desired support, automatically and effectually prevents any prolapse; while the handle of the faucet, projecting forward, between the limbs, may be manipulated with the greatest ease in controlling the flow of water; and, being seated on a warm cushion, the patient experiences a pleasant, soothing sensation, which completely allays any nervousness.

Moreover, realizing the immense advantage to be obtained by attacking the germs of disease in their chief breeding place, an antiseptic preparation is introduced into the water used in this remedial process, which completely and speedily destroys the germs of disease; but although so potent in its action upon micro-organic life, it is perfectly harmless, even though a hundred times the necessary quantity should be forced into the intestinal canal. But it is not alone a germ destroyer, for it possesses admirable tonic properties, which act upon the muscular coat of the colon and speedily restores it to its normal condition.

Defecation, or the expulsion of waste substance from the bowel is accompanied by the contraction of the circular fibres of the said muscular coat, but when constipation has existed for any length of time, the accumulated matter adhering to the walls of the colon renders that organ partially, if not wholly rigid, hence the difficulty of evacuation; consequently, through disuse, the muscles become to a certain extent atrophied, and require stimulation to resume their natural function even after the colon has been cleansed. It is largely owing to the use of this antiseptic "tonic" that the "Cascade Treatment" has been so successful in cases of obstinate constipation, as by its use the intestine speedily regains tone and power.

I unhesitatingly assert that if the colon be regularly cleansed and disinfected by this means, any bacilli or bacteria that may have obtained a lodgment in the system will be quickly destroyed and expelled--it cannot be otherwise.

And once the germs of disease are destroyed and their chief breeding place kept clean by this simple process, and the re-absorption of poisonous liquid waste into the system thus prevented, Nature, the great physician, will speedily assert itself and effect a restoration to health.

NOTE.

If the water is not readily expelled do not attempt to force it out by straining. Instead, flatten in the abdomen by forcibly contracting the abdominal muscles.

PART IV.

HOW TO USE IT.

Having endeavored to show the true nature of disease, the rational method of treating it, and the superiority of the "Cascade" over all previously existing methods for carrying the treatment into effect, it may be well to explain the actual manner of using the "Cascade."

In the first place, the reservoir should be thoroughly washed out with slightly warm water, to get. rid of the factory dust. At one time it was the practice to cleanse them all thoroughly before fitting them, but purchasers got the impression that they had been used by other persons, so it was decided to abandon that practice and send them out with the dust of the factory in them, in proof of their newness.

Having cleansed the reservoir, the faucet should be shut off and a level teaspoonful of the antiseptic tonic dissolved in a little warm water in a cup or glass and poured into the reservoir, which should then be completely filled with water as hot as the hand can comfortably bear; not to simply dip the fingers in and withdraw them, but so that you can immerse the hand and allow it to remain without discomfort. If tested with a thermometer the water should be from 100 to 105 degrees Fahr., but the hand is a safer guide, as it prevents any possible danger from a thermometer out of order, or mistaking a figure in a poor light. If tested by the hand you are absolutely safe, since water can he used twenty degrees hotter internally than externally, but in its passage from the body it would he painful to the external parts. Hot water is the best solvent for impacted faecal matter, and, on the other hand, water below the temperature of the body is likely to cause pain. If the hands are impervious to heat, an excellent plan is to test the water with the tip of the elbow, which is a most sensitive part of the body.

It is necessary that the reservoir should be absolutely full to insure the exclusion of air, as that is also likely to cause pain, and, in addition, its presence is likely to prevent the proper reception of the water, as, according to an established law in physics, two bodies cannot occupy the same space at the same time. For this reason it is advisable to solicit the bowels before taking the treatment, as, if even no faecal matter is expelled, pent-up gases are frequently liberated.

The reservoir having been filled as directed and the above directions carefully observed, the "Cascade" should be laid down and the "injection point" screwed in. It is then ready for use. Being all ready, the stick of rectal soap should be dipped in water--to moisten it--inserted in the rectum and withdrawn. This is simply to lubricate the passage and facilitate the admission of the "injection point." Then, standing in front of the seat on which the "Cascade" is lying (as if preparing to sit down), pass the left hand between the lower limbs and grasp the handle of the faucet, to guide the "injection point" into the rectum, and then carefully sit down upon the "Cascade." When the "injection point" has been completely introduced and you are comfortably seated, relax the muscles and allow the whole weight of the body to rest freely on the "Cascade," and turn on the faucet, partially at first, then, after a few seconds, turn it on fully and you will readily receive the water.

The most convenient place to use the "Cascade" is in the bathroom, placing it on the closet seat; or you will find the ordinary bedroom "commode" a suitable article for the purpose, but if neither of these are available, then any firm seat, such as a wooden-seated chair, will do, but taking care to have a vessel at hand in which to discharge the contents of the bowel.

As soon as the faucet is turned on and the water begins to flow into the body, proceed to practise the following movements: Commencing in the right groin; stroke firmly but gently, right across the pelvis, or lower edge of the abdomen, to the left groin, then directly upward with the hands to a point just above the umbilicus, or navel, then straight across the body and down to the right groin. These movements are directly over and along the course of the colon, and if they are made gently but firmly, the water will be assisted on its course. A study of the diagram of the digestive apparatus at the commencement of the book will be of great assistance in enabling you to understand the reason for and the method of these movements.

It sometimes happens that after a small quantity of water has been injected there is a strong desire to expel it, which is sometimes due to nervousness, induced by the novelty of the operation. If this be so, shut off the faucet at once and resist the inclination, when, in a few minutes, the desire will have passed away, then turn on the faucet again. Be sure to allow the full weight of the body to rest on the "Cascade," and have no fear. It is the weight of the body itself that furnishes the motive power and to ease up the pressure defeats the object.

As soon as all the water has entered that you feel it possible to receive, turn off the faucet, rise from the "Cascade," sit over the closet, or vessel, and allow the contents of the bowel to escape. At the same time repeat the stroking movement previously described, but this time reverse it, commencing in the right groin, up, across and down to the left groin. These movements have a three-fold object: they assist the water in its passage backward and forward, thus shortening the time of the treatment; they force along the accumulated matter in the colon with the current of water, and help to dislodge adherent matter from the walls of the colon.

As we proceed on the assumption that the colon is more or less impacted (which experience shows), we do not anticipate that more than two quarts will be received at the first treatment, but as the accumulations are removed by successive treatments, the capacity of the colon is increased, so that at the end of the second week enough should be received to completely fill the colon. The amount of water varies, of course, with the bulk of the individual, but the capacity of the colon, in the average well-grown adult, is about four quarts, but even in the case of a person below the average size, it may safely be assumed that three quarts of water are absolutely necessary for a successful treatment.

The presence of from three to four quarts of water in the body will naturally distend the abdomen and produce a little discomfort, but no apprehension of any harmful result need be entertained. Rest assured of this: it is absolutely impossible to rupture the colon, unless you were to use a force pump, and even then, before the point of rupture could be reached, the pain would be so intense that you would be compelled to desist. Again, as we have pointed out, the colon is a wonderfully elastic organ, and it would be an impossibility to distend it with water to the same extent that it is frequently distended by faecal accumulations.

Whenever pain is present during the treatment it is usually due to one of two things: either the water has not been sufficiently hot, or the reservoir has not been completely filled, but, if in spite of these precautions, pain should be present, it will be found advisable, after a small quantity of water has been injected (say from a pint to a quart) to shut off the faucet, rise from the "Cascade" and expel it; then, upon returning to the "Cascade," it will usually be found that the cleansing of the lower portions of the bowel has removed the trouble. The same method of procedure holds good when there is any difficulty in injecting the water. In cases where pain is persistent, even although all precautions are taken (although such are extremely rare), a decoction of anise seed made by steeping a tablespoonful of the seed in a pint of boiling water, added to the water used for flushing (omitting the antiseptic tonic), will act as an anodyne on the intestine, and completely subdue the pain.

The frequency with which the treatment is used will depend upon the nature of the trouble and the length of time it has existed. In the great majority of cases it is recommended to be used as follows when commencing the treatment: The first week use it every night; the second week every alternate night; after that use it twice a week, or as occasion seems to demand it. For the simple preservation of health, twice a week will be found amply sufficient. After using the "Cascade" it will be found extremely beneficial to inject from a half pint to a pint of cool water and retain it. This will be found not only a valuable rectal tonic, but an excellent diuretic as well, as it will pass off by way of the kidneys, cleansing and purifying those organs.

The "Cascade" should not be used within three hours after eating a full meal, as, if both the stomach and transverse colon are distended at the same time they press upon each other, and the stomach, being the more sensitive of the two, nausea is likely to be produced; but although (with the above proviso) the treatment can be used with benefit at any period during the twenty-four hours, yet, just before retiring at night is by far the best time to take it, for several reasons. Firstly, it is usually the most convenient time for the majority of people. Secondly, it invariably induces a good night's rest; for no sleeping potion can equal its effects in that direction. Thirdly, night is Nature's repairing season, when she is busy making good the ravages of the day--replacing the waste by building fresh tissue and by putting the system into a cleanly condition and purifying the blood current; at that season you are co-operating with Nature and may confidently expect, and will undoubtedly secure, the best results.

After using the "Cascade" it is quite possible that there may not be a movement of the bowels until late the following day. This must not be considered as evidence of constipation, but simply a lack of matter to discharge. In a perfectly natural condition of existence there should be at least two movements of the bowels during the day, but it must be remembered that the human system has acquired bad habits, and it will require some time before perfect conditions are re-established. If, however, from a half pint to a pint of hot water is sipped in the morning, certainly not less than half an hour before breakfast, it will stimulate the bowels to action, even though the "Cascade" had been used the night before, while its cleansing effect upon the stomach will assist the digestive functions in a marked degree.

It may be accepted as a truism that success invariably excites envy, therefore, it is but reasonable that the astounding results that have attended this method of treatment should have aroused a certain amount of antagonism. The hardy individual who dares to propose a new departure in the method of treating disease must be prepared to hear his theories ridiculed, his system denounced, and, possibly, his motives impugned. Consequently, it is not surprising that the "Cascade Treatment" has some objections urged against it.

The first objection I am confronted with is, "it is not natural." I willingly concede that point, and will add that neither is an obstructed and engorged colon natural.

We are living (in a large measure) an artificial life. In his barbaric state man obeyed the calls of nature without regard to time or place, and it is safe to assert that under those conditions an obstructed colon was an unknown quantity. But in deference to the demands of civilized life we disregard Nature's calls and defer the response until a convenient opportunity presents itself, and for this violation of natural law, a penalty is inflicted.

An obstructed colon, therefore, being itself unnatural, man is obviously justified in using the brains that Nature has endowed him with to cleanse it. An artificial limb is unnatural, but would the same objection hold good that because a man has had the misfortune to suffer amputation, he must, therefore, limp through life on crutches, rather than use the mechanical substitute that man's ingenuity has devised?

Common sense teaches us, and experience has amply confirmed the teaching, that flushing is not only the easiest, but the most effectual means of accomplishing this purpose; and it is unmistakably the most harmless, inasmuch as we use Nature's most simple and effective cleansing agency in the process--pure water. Sickness is in itself unnatural, and until the system can be restored to its natural condition reason plainly shows us that we must co-operate with Nature and assist in removing these impurities from the system, a task which our disregard of her warnings has prevented her from accomplishing. Cathartics simply excite the excretory processes, and stimulate Nature to a violent effort to expel them, the unnatural exertion being followed by a feeling of languor, for all purgative action is debilitating. Flushing, on the contrary, acts directly on the accumulated matter in the colon (which cathartics never do), and, instead of causing an unnatural excitation of any of the natural processes, it induces a calm, restful feeling and a sense of profound relief.

"It is a debilitating practice," the objectors urge. Here, again, I join issue. I am in a position to prove a decided negative.

I have the evidence of thousands of people to the contrary--people who have tested the treatment, and, setting aside the weight of testimony, even the most prejudiced mind must admit, that actual, personal experience is more to be relied on than unsupported theory.

Dr. Contrary--people said that his patients who had used the treatment for months, and even years, had steadily gained in strength and flesh all the time.

Another favorite objection is that "it causes the intestines to become weakened and dependent upon this unnatural method." To this I reply that it is a well known fact that at least fifty per cent, of people in civilized (?) communities are slaves to the purgative habit, the system refusing to fulfil its functions without this unnatural excitation; therefore, if dependence must be placed in something, we should unhesitatingly give the preference to water, as against cathartics, but the whole weight of evidence shows that the objection has no foundation in fact.

On this subject Dr. Forrest said: "Flushing the colon does not cause a weakening of the intestines. When this procedure is no longer necessary, owing to restored health, the intestines have also been restored and improved in tone and will carry on their functions unaided."

Dr. Stevens, who has used the treatment upon himself and patients for over twenty years, says that it in no wise interferes in his case with the normal movement of the bowels. To test it in this respect he has frequently discontinued its use for a week, with the result of a regular movement, as soon as enough faecal matter had accumulated to demand it.

He recommends flushing every two or three days as a preventive of disease. For over twenty years he has practiced flushing upon himself as a precaution, and, although now between seventy and eighty years old, since beginning its use he has never known a day of sickness.

It is contended by some people, including a percentage of physicians (who should know better), that the frequent use of this treatment will so stretch the colon that it will remain permanently distended. This argument is so totally opposed to physiological law, to say nothing of experience and common sense, that it is almost laughable. The veriest tyro in the matter of exercise knows that exercise develops a muscle; that repeated flexion and extension of the arm, for instance, will strengthen the muscles of that limb, not cause them to lose their contractibility. All muscle fibres are alike in structure, except that some are voluntary, others involuntary, but that difference is simply due to the difference in the source of nerve supply. There is no reason that can be shown why the muscles of the colon should lose their elasticity through exercise in contra-distinction to all the other muscles of the body, since they are not subjected to any extraordinary strain, the extreme tension only lasting for a few seconds, while as soon as the water commences to escape, relaxation follows, and, in addition, heat acts as a stimulant. The objection does not even merit serious consideration.

"It operates against peristalsis," we are told. I deny it, for the energy evinced by the intestine in expelling the water is proof of increased peristaltic vigor, if it is proof of anything. And even if it did suspend peristalsis for a few minutes, is it not a fact that other natural functions can be suspended for a much longer period, only to be resumed with unabated vigor?

Equally absurd, and destitute of foundation, in fact, is the objection frequently advanced that the washing of the interior surface of the colon is injurious; as it washes away the fluid that Nature secretes for the purpose of lubrication.

Where, in the name of common sense, do they get their authority for such a statement? Do they not know that such a contention is in direct opposition to physiological law? Does bathing the external surface of the body prevent the further excretion of perspiration; or bathing the eyes destroy the functions of the Meibomian glands? Does the drinking of water prevent any further discharge of saliva into the mouth, or of gastric juice into the stomach? If the washing away of a secretion destroyed the power of the secreting gland, human existence would be brief indeed.

The truth is that not one in ten thousand has any practical knowledge of the subject. They may possess a smattering, and in the endeavor to make it show to advantage, they draw upon their imagination to supply the deficiency. On the other hand, I have been making this subject a constant study for the past twenty years, having had experience in thousands of cases, and, therefore, contend that my opinion is of more value than that of the average man--whether physician or layman--and is at least entitled to respectful consideration.

Whether the practice of the treatment is to be persisted in will, of course, depend upon the nature and habits of the patient. If the pernicious habits that caused the trouble are not abandoned, a constant resort to the treatment will be necessary. If the patient is naturally of a costive habit, and has thoroughly weakened his intestines by a reckless and indiscriminate use of cathartics, it will require a long persistence in reformed habits before the weakened bowels will have gained sufficient strength to fulfil their functions normally.

It is advisable for elderly people to use it more or less continuously throughout life, for with advancing years the bowels naturally become less active, and this simple process offers a valuable means of assistance to flagging nature at the cost of little, if any, exertion; in fact, after a, little experience no more will be thought of using the "Cascade" than of taking a meal.

I would strictly impress on the minds of those who propose to give this treatment a trial that, like every other undertaking in life, thoroughness and persistence are absolutely indispensable to success. No great end was ever yet achieved except by hard work, conscientiousness and perseverance, and these three factors are in the highest degree necessary to restore health to a system from which it has long been estranged:

If a chronic, deep-seated disease can be cured in a year, by a home process, so simple that a child can understand and practise it, the individual so benefited should consider himself or herself most fortunate; and few will deny that the end in view--restoration to health--is a full and ample recompense for the thorough and persistent effort necessary to attain it. If it were a question of large pecuniary profit to the patient, it is scarcely necessary to say that every nerve would be strained to its utmost tension to bring the coveted prize within his grasp; yet here the reward is of infinitely greater value, a prize compared with which riches are as dross in comparison with gold. It is Health, without which the acquisition of Wealth, is well-nigh impossible, and its possession as profitless to the possessor as Dead Sea fruit.

I write thus strongly on this point because there is a large class of people who dabble in every new system of treatment projected, and toy with every medicinal device that is placed upon the market. They are the class from whom the patent medicine vendor draws his enormous annual profits. Like a bee in a garden of roses, they flit from one remedy to another, but, unlike that energetic and acquisitive insect, they do not gather the golden reward they are in search of--health. It is the purveyor of the nostrum that secures whatever there is of gold.

They seem to be utterly incapable of continuity of effort, and, unless they can discern a marked improvement within a week after commencing a fresh method of treatment, get discouraged and abandon it. To this class of people I say, in the most emphatic manner, that if they propose to give this great remedial process a trial and expect to derive benefit from it, that the cure rests entirely in their own hands.

They must persevere. They must be thorough. They must not expect miraculous results in a few days. Their diseased condition is the growth of months, perhaps years, and it is the height of unreasoning folly to expect to be cured in a few weeks. A merchant whose business has been crippled and who starts in to rebuild it, will consider himself an extremely fortunate man if, by watchful and untiring endeavor, he can restore it to a sound and healthy condition in a few years. Growth is necessarily slow--and this is especially the case with the human system. Nature will not be hurried. But of one thing they may rest assured, and that is that if they conscientiously and persistently practise this simple hygienic treatment they will find Nature a responsive and willing coadjutor.

"Heaven fights on the side of the strongest battalions," is a military aphorism, and Nature ranges herself on the side of the individual who co-operates with her most faithfully, who, in the struggle for the regaining of health, brings the greatest amount of determination and perseverence to the encounter.

What these irresolute dabblers in "medical fads" need most of all is to be inoculated with good, sound common sense, but until some method is discovered for the accomplishment of that psychological feat, they will continue to run hither and thither after every new remedy, dallying with all, and deriving benefit from none.

Here is the testimony of an intelligent man who realizes that the cure of a chronic disease must necessarily be a gradual process:

"I was a great sufferer from kidney disease of long standing. The doctors and the various remedies recommended for this complaint afforded me no relief. I have now used your treatment for nearly six months. It is working wonders. While I am not yet entirely cured, I am a great deal better than I was, and am sure, with the rate of progress made, in six months more I shall be entirely cured."

Perseverence in the treatment will achieve results that seem little short of miraculous to those accustomed to the "hit or miss" methods that have so long been in use. And best of all, the benefit attained will be permanent, for the system being thoroughly cleansed, and kept so, nothing but fresh, firm, healthy tissue is formed, so that after a year's conscientious treatment the person practising it will be practically a new being.

PART V.

PRACTICAL HYGIENE.

Of all the dangers by which we are menaced, none is so greatly to be apprehended as ignorance. This is especially true with reference to health. The majority of people fall easy victims to disease, simply through ignorance of the fundamental principles that govern health. It is because they do not rise superior to this ignorance concerning the health of their bodies that they become the prey of the unscrupulous charlatans who thrive upon the maladies of humanity, and the patent medicine vendors whose specious advertisements beguile them of their money. The humiliating part of it is that these same imposters (in a large majority of cases) possess but little more knowledge of these subjects than their dupes, but are absolutely devoid of conscientious scruples. It behooves every intelligent individual to see that this reproach is lifted from him. Knowledge is held to be a valuable possession in every department of life; but in no instance will it yield greater returns for the investment than in the field of hygiene--in learning how to keep well.

It must not be imagined that because the treatment previously described is such a wonderful curative and preventive of disease that nothing more is necessary that all other hygienic measures can be ignored. These bodies of ours were given us for a nobler purpose than to be the sport of our caprice or neglect. It is our duty to treat them as a divine trust.

There is no reason why any human being should die before eighty at least. With proper care the century mark should be reached in the majority of cases. This may sound like an extravagant assertion, but it is absolutely true. It all depends upon taking care of the human machine. Ask an engineer how long a locomotive would last if drawn at express speed every day, or if left standing idly on a siding! He will tell you that over work or disuse are fatal to mechanism, so far as its capacity for lasting is concerned. Well, the most finished product of man's handiwork in machinery cannot begin to compare with that wonderful, complex piece of mechanism--the human body; and if care will prolong the life of the lifeless machine, the veriest dullard cannot fail to perceive that the same rule applies with ten-fold force to the human organism, which possesses within itself the power of recuperation--a living machine, every atom of which is being daily replaced as fast as the friction of life disintegrates it. If the locomotive were capable of being reproduced in like manner--of having the daily waste of substance replaced during rest by proper attention to its needs--do you think its owners would ever allow it to wear or rust out? Would they not bend every energy to prolong its existence indefinitely? Most assuredly they would. And is the body, the earthly habitation of the real man, of less importance to himself than the creations of his own hands? Common sense says, "No!" But daily experience shows us that the bulk of humanity are far less careful of the earthly husk that shelters the divine ego than of the machinery that ministers to their wants. We repeat, there is no reason why man should not live to be a hundred, or even more, if only proper care be exercised. The hurry of modern life is fatal to the expectation of longevity, so also is over-indulgence in the pleasures of the table, which is one of the besetting sins of the present generation. If from childhood the care of the human body was made the subject of constant instruction, the second generation from now would see such a marked change in the personnel of the race as would astound even the most sanguine. What if a few less dollars were piled on each other? "Which is the more to be desired, a perfect, healthful physique, or a full purse?"

To preserve the body in health is an easy matter, if the individual will only bring the same thoughtful intelligence to bear on the subject that he does on the ordinary affairs of life. The natural agencies for the preservation of health are, as previously stated, Pure Water, Sunlight, Fresh Air, Diet and Exercise. he first three are furnished "without money and without price" by the all-wise mother, while the two last simply require a slight exertion of will power, tempered with intelligence.

Of the quintette of agencies mentioned above, water is one of the most important. Water is the original source of all animal life. From it the earliest species were evolved, and by the natural law of correlation, it continues to be one of the most important factors in sustaining existence. Water enters more largely into the composition of all organic substance than the majority of people dream of, and this is notably true of the human body. Few people realize that seventy per cent. of their earthly tenement consists of the fluid in which they perform their ablutions, yet such is the fact.

This important physiological truth should be carefully laid to heart, for it accentuates the vital necessity of imbibing a sufficient quantity of fluid daily to preserve the proportion in the system requisite for health! Water is the only known substance that possesses the power of permeating every cell and fibre of the living organism, without creating disturbance or irritation. Water is, in fact, an indispensable necessity for physical existence its excess or deficit creating abnormal conditions; but the latter is the more common condition. Being universally present in all the tissues of the body, water is the principal agent in the elimination of waste material from the body, according to Nature's plan--hence, for the preservation of health, every adult should drink from two to three quarts of water per day, certainly not less than two quarts. One of the remedial factors in the copious use of water in "flushing the colon" is that a liberal percentage of it is absorbed through the walls of the colon, directly into the circulation, thus increasing the amount in the tissues, and causing more fluid to pass through the kidneys--cleansing them.

Hot water is, in reality, a "natural scavenger," but its virtues are only imperfectly known. As a therapeutic agent it is almost without a peer, and yet it is so little used that it is practically a dead letter. Chemists are burning the midnight oil in their laboratories searching for new weapons with which to fight sepsis, while hot, boiled water, which is one of the best antiseptics in existence, is almost ignored. It may be asked why (if it is such an invaluable remedial agent) it is not more extensively used and advocated? In the first place, its merits are not generally known. In the second place, physicians who know of its value hesitate to prescribe it, for the reason that the majority of patients expect the doctor to prescribe drugs, and are disappointed if he does not. There is a tendency on the part of the majority of people to slight that which is near at hand and easily obtained, in favor of those things which are designated by mysterious titles, or are difficult of attainment. Man has been so long accustomed to regard with a species of awe the hieroglyphics on orthodox prescriptions, that he finds it difficult to dissociate from it the idea of talismanic power.

But to return to its uses. Hot water used as a stomach bath (see description in the appendix at end of book) is a valuable auxiliary in the preservation and restoration of health.

By its means the stomach is cleansed of mucous accumulations and particles of undigested food, thus enabling it to perform its functions satisfactorily. If, as is often the case (more especially with dyspeptics) undigested food remains in the stomach, it ferments, causing what is known as sour stomach, and is productive of many evils. If we keep the ferment out of the stomach by occasionally washing it, and prevent the generation of foul gases in the colon, by regularly flushing it, the bile will effectually prevent any fermentation in the intestines; and with the body in this cleanly condition, sickness is well-nigh impossible. But there are external applications of water, which are equally important for the preservation of health, and first and foremost is the bath.

It is a matter of authentic history that the most highly enlightened and prosperous people of the world have been celebrated for their devotion to the bath as a means of securing health and vigor as a means of curing disease, and preventing it, by promoting the activity of the skin. The excavations at Pompeii show the devotion of the people to luxurious bathing. The Romans are famous to this day for the magnificence of their lavatories and the universal use of them by the rich and poor alike. In Russia the bath is general, from the Czar to the poorest serf, and through all Finland, Lapland, Sweden and Norway, no hut is so destitute as not to have its family bath. Equally general is the custom in Turkey, Egypt and Persia, among all classes from the Pasha down to the poorest camel driver. Pity it is that we cannot say as much for the people of our own country.

Most people are familiar with the aphorism, "cleanliness is next to godliness," a statement that by implication relegates cleanliness to the second place, but we would transpose this stated sequence of conditions, and assign the premier position to cleanliness; for we contend that purity of soul presupposes purity of body. It is true that we sometimes find a "jewel in an Ethiop's ear," but it is the exception that proves the rule.

But it is not from the moral standpoint that we wish to consider the subject of physical cleanliness, but from the hygienic. How few people there are who are really physically clean! The outward semblance of cleanliness too frequently poses as the real article. Even people who pride themselves on their cleanliness are frequently guilty of the unclean practice of sleeping in the underwear they have worn during the day, and would feel aggrieved if their unclean habit was called by its right name. Yet, what can be more repulsive to the truly cleanly individual than the retention, next the body, of garments saturated with the constant exhalations from the system? Those who think this a trifling matter, should turn their underwear wrong side outward (after removing it) when retiring for the night, and in the morning shake it thoroughly, when they will receive an object lesson in the form of a cloud of dried effete matter, consisting largely of particles of the epidermis, removed by abrasion, through the friction of the clothing. This, being visible, appeals to the sense of sight; but gives no evidence of the gaseous and liquid refuse matter which was deposited in the material, and has been allowed to evaporate by the removal of the clothing. Thus we may see how many so-called cleanly people fall hopelessly short of true cleanliness. If the individual keeps the surface of the body clean, by frequent ablutions, the evil is lessened; but how many people bathe the body daily? As Hamlet says: "It is a custom more honored in the breach than the observance." Among the white races of the earth, the English are the greatest devotees of the daily tub, to which custom their ruddy complexions are largely due; but Japan is preeminently in the lead in the matter of daily bathing, for it is doubtful if there could be found in the land of the "little brown people" a single individual who does not bathe the whole body daily, unless physically incapacitated.

The skin is such an important excretory organ that the importance of keeping its innumerable infinitesimal outlets free from obstruction cannot be overestimated. As the structure of the skin may not be understood by the average reader, we will briefly describe this wonderful depurating organ, that the paramount importance of its functions may be properly appreciated.

The skin consists of two layers, the derma, or true skin, and the epidermis, or cuticle. It is the principal seat of the sense of touch, and on the surface of the upper layer are the sensitive papillae, which receive and respond to impressions; and within, or imbedded beneath it, are organs with special functions, viz., the sweat glands, hair follicles and sebaceous glands. Its value as a means of depuration is incalculable, as by it, vast quantities of the aqueous and gaseous refuse matter is conveyed from the body. By the aid of a four diameter magnifying glass applied to the skin of the palm of the hand, the curiously inclined will observe that it is divided into fine ridges, which are punctured regularly with minute holes. These are the mouths of the sweat glands, and generally known as the pores of the skin. Their function is to bring moisture to the surface of the skin; which is secreted from the blood, and chemical analysis reveals the fact that this moisture is always more or less loaded with worn-out and effete matter. It is estimated that there are 3,800 of these glands in each square inch of skin, and that their total length, in an ordinary person, if placed end to end, would be ten miles. Then there are the sebaceous, or oil glands, which oil the skin and keep it flexible. Now, as the processes of destruction and upbuilding are perpetually going on in the body, and the skin being one of the principal avenues by which the refuse is removed, the vital necessity of keeping this organ perfectly clean becomes apparent at once; for this refuse matter, if retained in the system, acts as a poison, and furnishes food for disease germs to feed upon.

It has been demonstrated by experiment upon dogs from which the hair had been shorn, that a coat of varnish applied to the body (thus effectually closing the pores), will cause death in a very short while. No better object lesson could be given of the imperative necessity of keeping the skin perfectly clean, if you wish to enjoy good health.

It is an easy matter to keep all these miles of tubing in a perfectly natural and active condition, by a strict observance of the fundamental principle--cleanliness. Bathe the body daily, complete immersion, if practicable; if this is not possible, then sponge the body thoroughly, all over; but if both methods are rendered out of the question by circumstances, then adopt the best substitute, namely, vigorous friction with a coarse towel.

We know it will be urged that the majority of people have not the time or convenience for this daily process; but when sickness overtakes them, they have to find time to submit to medical treatment, and in this, as in other matters of everyday life, the cleanly individual who is thoroughly in earnest, will "find a way, or make it."

As to the temperature of the bath, that must, to a great extent, depend upon the conditions of life, and the predisposition and susceptibility of the individual; but the cold bath should always be employed in preference to the warm bath, when conditions permit. The cold bath is a powerful stimulant to the sympathetic nervous system. and as that is the great regulator of nutrition, the value of cold bathing to those afflicted with digestive disturbances will be readily understood, since all the digestive and assimilative processes are quickened by it. The glands of the stomach secrete more hydrochloric acid on account of this stimulus, and a better quality of gastric juice being thus formed, not only is the digestion improved, but the system is better enabled to resist microbic invasion. The cold bath also stimulates the vaso-motor system, which regulates the circulation, by contracting and dilating the vessels, and increases the activity of the capillaries or small blood vessels. It thus increases the resisting power of the skin, by enabling it to reheat the surface after a chill, and this is the reason why people who habitually use the cold bath are practically proof against "colds."

People employed in sedentary occupations are especially benefited by the cold bath, but should employ a hot bath for three or four minutes beforehand. It is also especially beneficial to women, as, being an excellent nerve tonic, it successfully combats all forms of nervous weakness, and is an admirable preventive of hysteria.

Children under seven years of age do not bear the application of cold water very well, and it is advisable not to use the water at a lower temperature than 700 Fahr., and to employ friction constantly while administering it; but after that age the temperature may be gradually lowered. In old age the neutral bath, from 75 to 850 Fahr. will be found the best for general use, accompanied by friction.

The bath, to be thoroughly beneficial, should be taken at one of the three following portions of the day, immediately upon rising, about ten o'clock, or just before going to bed. The early morning bath is, however, immeasurably the best, and if cold, will be found a wonderful aid in promoting health and vigor, and being such a necessity, especially in the preservation of health, and the constant practice of it, strongly urged, we append the following useful suggestions for guidance:

A full meal should not be taken in less than half an hour after bathing. Nor should a bath be taken in less than an hour and a half after eating a full meal.

You can bathe with impunity in cold water when the body is perspiring freely, as long as the breathing is not disturbed, nor the body exhausted by over-exertion.

Never bathe in cool or cold water when the body is cold. First restore warmth by exercise.

Always wet the head before taking a plunge bath, and the chest also, if the lungs are weak.

In cases of sickness, where it becomes necessary to assist Nature in ridding the system of impurities through the medium of the sweat glands, the "wet sheet pack" will be found invaluable. It is usually regarded by those imperfectly acquainted, with its action as simply the chief factor in a sweating process, but it is more than that. Not only does it open up the pores and soften the scales of the skin, but it "draws" the morbid matter from the interior of the body, through the surface to the pores. It is of immense value in all cases of fever, especially bilious fever.

It should be borne in mind that "flushing the colon" should always precede the use of the "pack."

If any one doubts the purifying efficacy of this process he can have a "demonstration strong" by the following experiment: Take any man in apparently fair health, who is not accustomed to daily bathing, who lives at a first-class hotel, takes a bottle of wine at dinner, a glass of brandy and water occasionally, and smokes from three to six cigars per day. Put him in a pack and let him soak one or two hours. On taking him out the intolerable stench will convince all persons present that his blood and secretions were exceedingly befouled and that a process of depuration is going on rapidly.

Full directions for the use of the pack will be found at the end of this work.

It will be necessary to take into consideration the vitality of the patient and regulate the temperature of the sheet accordingly. The best time to use it is about ten in the morning, or nine in the evening.

The Turkish bath (see last page) is another important factor in treating disease, also the hot foot bath, for all disturbances of the circulation, cramps, spasms and affections of the head and throat. Hot fomentations, which draw the blood to the seat of pain, thereby raising the local temperature and affording relief, and wet bandages for warming and cooling purposes will likewise be found valuable aids.

Humanity at large has never estimated water at its true value, yet all the gifts in Pandora's fabled box could never equal that one inestimable boon of the Creator to the human race. Apart from its practical value, there is nothing in all the wide domain of Nature more beautiful, for in all its myriad forms and conditions it appeals equally to the artistic sense. In the restless ocean, now sleeping tranquilly in opaline beauty beneath the summer sun, now rising in foam-crested mountainous waves beneath the winter's biting blast, its sublimity awes us, In the mighty river, rolling majestically on its tortuous course, impatient to unite itself with mother ocean, its resistless energy fascinates us. In the gigantic iceberg, with its translucent sides of shimmering green, its weird grandeur enthralls us. In the pearly dew drop, glittering on the trembling leaf, or the hoar frost, sparkling like a wreath of diamonds in the moon's silvery rays: in the brawling mountain torrent, or the gentle brook--meandering peacefully through verdant meadows, in the mighty cataract or the feathery cascade, in the downy snowflake, or the iridescent icicle--in each and all of its many witching forms it is beautiful beyond compare. But its claims to our admiration rest not alone upon its ever varying beauty. When consumed with thirst, what beverage can equal a draught of pure, cold water? In sickness its value is simply incalculable especially in fevers; in fact, the famous lines of Sir Walter Scott, in praise of woman, might be justly transposed in favor of water to read thus:

"When pain and sickness wring the brow, A health-restoring medium thou."

And, if we admire it for its beauty and esteem it as a beverage, how inconceivably should these feelings be intensified by the knowledge that its remedial virtues are in nowise inferior to its other qualities!

The next in importance of the great health agencies is Fresh Air. Perhaps we ought to class it as the most important, for although people have been known to live for days without water, yet without air their hours would be quickly numbered. Air is a vital necessity to the human organism, and the fresher the better--it cannot be too fresh. The oxygen gas in the air is the vitalizing element. The blood corpuscles when they enter the lungs through the capillaries are charged with carbonic acid gas (which is a deadly poison), but when brought into contact with the oxygen, for which they have a wonderful affinity, they immediately absorb it, after ejecting the carbonic acid gas. The oxygen is at once carried to the heart, and by that marvelous pumping machine sent bounding through the arteries to contribute to the animal heat of the body.

When it is taken into account that the lungs of an average sized man contain upwards of six hundred millions of minute air cells, the surface area of which represents many thousands of square feet, the danger of exposing such a vast area of delicate tissue to the action of vitiated air can be readily estimated. No matter how nutritious the food may be that is taken into the stomach, no matter how perfect the processes of digestion and assimilation are, the blood cannot be vitalized without fresh air.

It is estimated that the blood is pumped through the lungs at the rate of eight hundred quarts per hour, and that during that period it rids itself of about thirty quarts of carbonic acid gas, and absorbs about the same amount of oxygen. Think for a moment of the madness of obstructing this interchange of elements which is perpetually going on and on which life depends!

It is more especially during the hours of sleep that fresh, pure air is needed, for that is when Nature is busiest, repairing and building up, and calls for larger supplies of oxygen to keep up the internal fires, but her efforts at repairing waste are rendered futile if you diminish the supply of the vitalizing element and compel her to use over again the refuse material she has already cast off.

The late Prof. Willard Parker, in a lecture delivered before a class of medical students, made a very forcible illustration of how the air of a room was vitiated, in the following impressive words: "If, gentlemen, instead of air you suppose this room filled with pure, clean water, and that instead of air you were exhaling twenty times a minute a pint of milk, you can see how soon the water, at first clear and sparkling, would become hazy and finally opaque; the milk diffusing itself rapidly through the water, you will thus be able, also, to appreciate how, at each fresh inspiration you would be taking in a liquid that grew momentarily more impure. Were we able to see the air as we see the water, we would at once appreciate how thoroughly we are contaminating it, and that unless there be some vent for the air thus vitiated, and some opening large enough to admit a pure supply of this very valuable material, we will be momentarily poisoning ourselves, as surely as if we were taking sewage matter into our stomachs." Don't leave the matter of a good supply of air to servants. See to it yourself and see that you are not robbed of it. It would be better to trust your eating to an attendant than your breathing. Do that yourself.

In spite of the amount of literature devoted to sanitary matters, it is astonishing how little is understood of the principles of ventilation, and its supreme importance to the general welfare. We do not, of course, refer to ventilation in its broadest scientific sense, such as the securing of an adequate air supply in large auditoriums, for it is a melancholy fact that even our prominent architects not only display a pitiably deficient grasp of that phase of the subject, but of the simple, yet fundamental principles of the science, which every intelligent adult should be familiar with. How many heads of families, for instance, can intelligently ventilate a sleeping room? They will open a window for a few minutes in the morning, without opening the door also, to create a current, and think that is amply sufficient to displace the accumulated carbon dioxide and other substances inimical to health. No wonder so many people are tormented by bad dreams! In sleeping apartments the bed should be in the center of the room--never near a wall. A current of air should be maintained, but without a draught upon the bed. It is better to open the window two inches at the bottom, and the same distance at the top, than to have it open for a foot either at the top or bottom only. If, through inclemency of the weather, or other causes, the window can only be opened for a few minutes, then by waving the door back and forth rapidly ten or a dozen times, the displacement of the vitiated air will be infinitely more rapid and thorough. Considering the length of time that is spent in the sleeping apartment, the paramount importance of a constant supply of fresh air is readily perceived. No matter how perfect digestion and assimilation may be, if the blood is not thoroughly oxygenated, the best of foods fail of their intended effect. Even the least fastidious would object to drinking water that had been used for washing purposes by others; yet it is quite as objectionable to breathe air that is charged with the waste products of bodies that may even be diseased. It is impossible to overestimate the importance of ventilation.

Better let in cold air and put on more bedclothes, as long as you do not sleep in a draught.

Oxygen keeps up the animal heat of the body, and you can really keep warmer in a room with plenty of fresh air than in a close room where the air is vitiated.

But in the sick room fresh air is of paramount importance, not only for the patient, but for the attendants, who are otherwise compelled to inhale the poisonous exhalations from the diseased body.

Let no consideration blind you, either in sickness or in health, to the imperative necessity of plenty of fresh air.

The next great natural agency, and one to which scant attention is paid, compared with its hygienic importance, is Light, but more especially Sunlight.

Light is essential to life. If by some monstrous cataclysm the sun was suddenly extinguished, it is impossible to conceive the misery that would follow. In the event of such a fearful calamity it would require but a very short time to depopulate the earth. We repeat, light is a necessity of existence, and it behooves us all to allow it free access to our dwellings. What if it does bleach carpets and draperies! Its beneficent effects are not to be measured by yards of wool and silk. Love of light is as instinctive as the aversion to darkness. Plants growing in a dark cellar, where but one struggling ray of light enters, will instinctively grow in the direction of that ray. It is questionable whether defective lighting is not productive of as much physical deterioration in the crowded tenement districts as defective ventilation--certainly it is only secondary in degree. Light is necessary. Light is free to all, and why human beings endowed with reason should attempt to exclude it from their dwellings is a thing that passes comprehension. Give the light free access to your dwelling. "Let there be light," is as imperative now as when the fiat went forth at the dawn of creation.

But Sunlight is the great health-giving agent. The sun is the great source of life. Its rays stimulate the growth of every living organism, and there is no doubt but they exert a chemical action upon living tissue with which we are as yet but imperfectly acquainted. This fact has been recognized of late years, hence our winter resorts are liberally supplied with sun parlors, in which those in quest of health may enjoy the rejuvenating effect of solar heat without exposing themselves to the inclemency of wintry weather. This is a revival of an old Roman custom, for the more opulent of that nation had sun baths on the roofs of their dwellings. Sunshine is as necessary to robust, vigorous health as either air or water. Then seize the full enjoyment of it whenever opportunity offers! It is a stimulant and tonic that has no superior. Go forth into the sunlight on every possible occasion! It is one of Nature's greatest therapeutic agents, and she bestows it ungrudgingly, without money and without price. If you are wise you will avail yourself of her bounty.

Do not be afraid to let the sunlight penetrate your dwellings, especially the morning sun. Thrifty housewives are prone to regard the actions of the sun's rays on their carpets and draperies as disastrous in the extreme, but its exclusion from their dwelling is far more disastrous to the health of the inmates. There is, of course, a happy medium in all things, and, therefore, it is not necessary to have the sun's rays streaming in through every door and window during the whole day; but the entire dwelling should be (as far as possible) thrown open to the vivifying beams of old Sol for a couple of hours in the morning, which at the same time will thoroughly ventilate the building. There is more virtue in sunlight than most people are aware of. Its bactericidal effects are only just beginning to be understood; but if you desire a healthful dwelling, let God's bright sunshine freely and frequently penetrate every corner of it.

It is astonishing how few people there are who properly estimate the hygienic value of the sun's rays. A valuable lesson on this point may be learned by observing the lower animals, none of which ever neglect an opportunity to bask in the sun And the nearer man approaches to his primitive condition the more he is inclined to follow the example of the animals. It is a natural instinct which civilization has partially destroyed in the human race.

The effect of sunshine is not merely thermal, to warm. and raise the heat of the body; its rays have chemical and electric functions. As a clever physician lately explained, it is more than possible that sunshine produces vibrations and changes of particles in the deeper tissues of the body, as effective as those of electricity. Many know by experience that the relief it affords to wearing pain, neuralgic and inflammatory, is more effective and lasting than that of any application whatever.

Those who have faceache should prove it for themselves, sitting in a sunny window where the warmth falls full on the cheek.

For nervous debility and insomnia the treatment of all others is rest in sunshine. Draw the bed to the window and let the patient lie in the sun for hours. There is no tonic like it--provided the good effects are not neutralized by ill-feeling. To restore a withered arm, a palsied or rheumatic limb, or to bring a case of nervous prostration up speedily, a most efficient part of the treatment would be to expose the limb or the person as many hours to direct sunlight as the day would afford. With weak lungs let the sun fall on the chest for hours. If internal tumor or ulceration is suspected, let the sun burn through the bear skin directly on the point of disease for hours daily. There will be no doubt left in the mind that there is a curative power in the chemical rays of the sun.

For the chilliness which causes blue hands and bad color, resort to the sun; let it almost blister the skin, and the circulation will answer the attraction. It is a finer stimulous than wine, electricity or massage, and we are on the verge of great therapeutic discoveries concerning it.

Some years ago a London surgeon, by using the sun's rays (presumably with a lens), removed a wine mark from a lady's face, and destroyed a malignant growth in the same way.

Says Dr. Thayer, of San Francisco:

"During a practice of more than a quarter of a century I have found no caustic or cautery to compare with solar heat in its beneficial results. Unlike other caustics, it can be applied with safety on the most delicate tissues and the system receives this treatment kindly. The irritation and inflammation following are surprisingly slight and of short duration, the pain subsiding immediately on removal of the lens. There is a curative power in the chemical rays of the sun yet unexplained."

Women especially need to make systematic trial of the sun's healing and rejuvenating rays. The woman who wants a cheek like a rose should pull her sofa pillows into the window and let the sun blaze first on one cheek and then on the other, and she will gain color warranted not to wash off.

Thus it will be seen that the curative properties of sunlight are in nowise overestimated, but in cases of sickness its beneficial action is purely supplementary. The system must first be thoroughly cleansed by "flushing the colon," then, the ground work of improvement being laid, Fresh Air and Sunlight will prove themselves worthy and efficient colleagues in the task of restoring health.

Singly, each is of intrinsic value, but inadequate to cope with disease single-handed (although they may mitigate it), but combined they form a Trinity so powerful that disease can never successfully oppose them.

The other two factors in Nature's great Health curriculum, namely, Exercise and Diet, will be considered under separate headings.

PART VI.

EXERCISE.

Motion is life. The health of both body and mind depend upon it. Inaction means stagnation, a condition fatal to health. Hence the necessity of exercise.

As before stated, disuse is as fatal to a piece of machinery as excessive use; in fact, it is far more likely to rust out than to wear out. Activity is essential to life and health and can never be prejudicial, provided that moderation is observed and the muscular system not strained or overworked.

There are thousands of miles of minute tubing in the human body--the arterioles, veins, capillaries and lymphatic vessels. They ramify through every portion of the body tissues, the first carrying the vitalized blood for nourishment of the parts, the second returning the impure blood, charged with the waste of the structures, the third being the intermediate stage between the first and second, while the fourth and last, the lymphatic vessels, collect the surplus nutrition and return it to the circulation. In addition the lymphatics assist in the conveyance of effete matter. Whenever disease germs are present in the system, they first manifest themselves in the lymph, but this fluid being densely populated with phagocyctes (white blood corpuscles), the micro-organisms are speedily destroyed, if the body is in a healthy, vigorous condition.

In view of the vital character of the fluids, activity of motion is indispensable for the best performance of their separate functions and exercise supplies the desired stimulus. Whenever a muscle is contracted the blood is wholly or partially expelled from it proportionately to the force of the contraction, and in its escape it carries with it the waste material; but as soon as the muscle is relaxed fresh blood from the arterial supply re-enters the structure, bearing fresh nutrition.

By a wise provision of Nature, the amount of nutrition supplied is always in excess of the waste products removed; that is, all things being equal, so that the more exercise a part is subjected to the more nutrition it receives. This explains the unusual development of certain parts of the body which are called into excessive use in certain occupations. But this unsymmetrical development is a thing to be avoided, as it is usually productive of certain deformities, such as stoop shoulders and certain peculiarities of gait, which are plainly noticeable in men employed in certain avocations.

The reason for this is perfectly simple, and may be expressed in two words--unequal nutrition--for the muscles that are unduly exercised appropriate the nutriment that should be equally distributed, so that the neglected muscles become weakened and stiff. Hence, any system of exercises designated to develop the body should be so arranged as to call into play every muscle in the individual, thus insuring harmonious development in every direction.

Muscular activity stimulates all the functions of the body. It has a most beneficial effect upon all the vital processes, digestion, assimilation and nutrition. The digestive powers work more briskly to prepare the needed nourishment, and the blood circulates more rapidly to carry the material for repair to the parts that need it, so that by moderate physical exercise, judiciously distributed, the whole body is built up and strengthened, and the result is a suppleness of frame and a clearness of head that makes life indeed worth living.

To the invalid it is, of course, idle to talk of active exercise, but there are certain forms of passive exercise accessible to such people. Massage, for instance, which, judiciously administered, will do for the sick, in a modified degree, what active exercise does for the comparatively well. It will stimulate the circulation in the deeper tissues, and set the various fluids of the body moving in a beneficial manner. There is also a mild form of active exercise which may be practised by those who have the misfortune to be confined to bed, and that is by tensing the muscles; such as clenching the hands and contracting the toes, also by gentle contraction of the arms and legs alternately.

But one of the most important factors in quickening and stimulating the movement of the fluids is exercising the lungs, and that can be accomplished with a fair measure of success even by the bed-ridden. Every time the chest cavity is emptied by the expiration of the breath a partial vacuum is created which exerts a tremendous suction power. It is one of the principal forces concerned in the return of the venous blood to the heart, but it also exerts a like effect upon the lymphatic current, hence deep breathing is a valuable exercise for those unable to take any other.

In commencing the development of the body by any system of physical culture, the first and most important thing to do is to develop the lungs. Good lungs and good digestion go together. Before food can be assimilated it must undergo oxygenation, which is neither more nor less than chemical combustion. For this oxygen is necessary, which, uniting with the carbon of the food, results in oxidation, and as the amount of oxygen inhaled depends upon the capacity of the lungs, it will readily be seen how much depends upon those organs. We cannot inhale too much oxygen, while we can take too much food; therefore, the greater the lung capacity the better the digestion.

We referred to the suction power of the empty chest cavity and its stimulating effect upon the fluids of the body. Now, the greater the lung capacity the greater the chest expansion and the vacuum produced by expiration; consequently the stimulating effect upon the fluids is correspondingly augmented.

Test your lungs by inhaling a full breath--inflate them to their full capacity--if it makes you dizzy you are in danger and should proceed at once to strengthen them. The following simple exercises will speedily result in improvement and are easy to practice:

HOW TO EXERCISE THE LUNGS.

1. When in the open air, walk erect, head up, chin drawn in, shoulders thrown back, thoroughly inflate the lungs and retain the air for a second or two, then expel it gently. Practice this several times a day, and if your employment keeps you in, make time and go out.

2. The first thing in the morning and the last thing at night, when you have nothing on but your underclothing, stand with your back against the wall and fill the lungs to their utmost capacity, then, retaining the breath gently tap the chest all over with the open hands. Do this regularly every morning and night, gently at first, but gradually increasing the length of time for holding the breath and the force of the blows as the lungs grow stronger.

3. Stand upright, heels touching, toes turned out. Place the hands on the hips, the fingers resting on the diaphragm, the thumbs in the soft part of the back. Now, inflate the lungs and force the air down into the lower back part of the lungs, forcing out the thumbs. Do this half a dozen times at first, gradually increasing the number. Women seldom use this part of the lungs--tight dresses and corsets prevent them.

4. While in the same position, fill the upper part of the lungs full, then force the air down into the lower part of the lungs and back again by alternately contracting the upper and lower muscles of the chest. Do this repeatedly, for, besides being a good lung developer, it is an excellent exercise for the liver.

5. Stand erect, the arms hanging close by the sides, then slowly raise the arms until they are in the same position, at the same time gradually taking in a full breath until the lungs are completely filled, then, after holding the breath for a few seconds, gradually lower the arms, at the same time gradually expelling the breath. After doing this a few times while the lungs are full raise and lower the arms several times quickly.

6. Hold the arms straight out, then slowly throw them back behind you as far as possible, at the same time taking a full breath, then bring them slowly back to the front, as at first, expelling the breath while doing so. Do this several times, then fully inflate the lungs, and while holding the breath move the arms backward and forward, in the same way, but quickly. It is important to inflate and empty the lungs fully and completely during this exercise.

COMBINATION LUNG AND MUSCLE EXERCISES.

7. First rotate the right arm in a circle, downward in front of you a few times, then reverse the movement. Next, thrust the shoulder back as far as it will go and rotate the arm in the same manner. Follow with the left arm in the same manner, then both alternately, but at the same time relax the arms completely, allowing them to become perfectly limp, at the same time filling and emptying the lungs completely.

8. Lie flat on the floor, face downward, with the elbows bent and the palms of the hands flat on the floor by the sides, body fully extended. Then, keeping the body perfectly rigid, raise it up by the muscles of the arms alone, until it only rests on the arms and toes, then lower the body gradually until the chest touches the floor, at the same time exercising the lungs to their fullest extent. This may be practiced on a bed or couch to commence with, and should be taken slowly at first, until it can be done half a dozen times without discomfort.

9. Stand with the lungs completely and force the air down into the lower

part of the lungs. Then, keeping the lower limbs perfectly stiff, with muscles tensed, bend the body forward from the middle of the trunk and while doing this empty the lungs quickly. Then straighten up again, at the same time filling the lungs. This should be repeated from 6 to 12 times. Then repeat the operation, but bending backward instead of forward, paying careful attention to the emptying and filling of the lungs. Then, with the lungs full and breath retained, move the body backward and forward quickly several times.

10. Retaining the same position as in last exercise, move the upper part of the body to the right a few times, then a few times to the left, after each movement returning to the upright position. Then move in the same manner from right to left, alternately. Study and you will readily understand the nature of these movements, which not only benefit the lungs, but impart grace and suppleness to the body.

11. Still retaining the attitude press the arms and elbows forward as far as possible, at the same time expelling the breath; then press them backward as far as possible to force them, at the same time inflating the lungs to their fullest extent.

ARM AND FINGER EXERCISES.

Completely relax the muscles of the fingers and hands, letting the hands hang limply from the wrists, then shake them up and down and from side to side, as if cracking a whip. Then rotate them from the wrists. These movements should all be made with great rapidity, the hands being rendered as near lifeless as possible.

12. Next, with the upper part of the arm held out at a right angle from the body, and the forearm hanging downward, completely relax the muscles of the elbow. Then shake and rotate the whole of the forearm in the same manner as described for the hands.

13. Allow the arms to hang by the side, now press the shoulder as far back as it will go, then as high as it will go, then forward as far as it will go, and drop it again, then rotate it several times. Do the same with the left, then both together. Strike out with the right hand, tightly clenched, then the left, then both together. Repeat horizontally, right and left, then straight up

overhead, then down by the sides.

EXERCISES FOR THE NECK.

14. The principal thing to be observed is to keep the body rigid and use the muscles of the neck only. It is a most valuable exercise and should be carefully and faithfully practiced.

15. Now, without bending the knees, bend the body forward as far as you can several times, then backward several times, then to each side successively. Make bending movements several times in each direction, and be careful not to relax the muscles other than those of the hips; and to conclude the exercise rotate the hips round and round.

16. Relax the muscles of the right leg, keeping all the other muscles firmly tensed. Then swing the leg from the hip joint, like a pendulum, backward and forward. Try to do this without support, balanced on the one leg, as it materially assists in developing the muscles. Then repeat with the left leg. Next, relax the muscles of the leg from the knee downward, keeping the muscles of the thigh rigid, and swing the leg backward and forward from the knee only, and increase the number of movements each day, as the muscles gain strength and you gain experience.

ANKLE AND FOOT EXERCISE.

17. Stand upright, holding yourself firmly and stiffly, then raise yourself up and down on your toes.

WHOLE BODY EXERCISE.

1. Raise the arms above the head, alongside the ears, then bring them down with a steady sweep, without bending the knees, until the fingers touch the floor. Be sure to relax the muscles of the neck and allow the head to hang.

2. Place the hands upon the breast and drop the head backward, a little to one side, then bend the body backward as far as possible.

3. Curve the right arm above the head, toward the left shoulder, and allow

the weight of the body to rest on the left leg, the right foot being carried slightly outward. Allow the body to bang down as far as possible on the left side, without straining too much. Then verse the movement.

STRETCHING.

Is quite a luxury, but few people know how to do it.

Stand upright in position, then raise raise yourself on the tips of your toes and try your best to touch the ceiling. You will appreciate this exercise as a relaxation.

THE ART OF STANDING PROPERLY.

Is only imperfectly understood by the majority of people, and yet it is the key to a graceful carriage, an accomplishment that most people desire to possess, especially ladies. Observe the difference between the correct and the incorrect methods.

THE ART OF GRACEFUL WALKING.

Is the natural sequence of correct attitude in standing and may be readily acquired by attention. Stand against the wall, with the heels, limbs, hips, shoulders and head all touching and draw the chin inward to the chest. When in this position you will find it uncomfortable, mainly because it is incorrect. Gently free yourself from the wall by swaying the body forward, from the ankles only, keeping the heels touching. You will then be in the correct position, and should walk off, carefully maintaining it. This exercise, if constantly practiced, will give you an easy and graceful carriage that will be the envy of your less fortunate acquaintances.

In the foregoing list of exercises we have carefully omitted all those requiring apparatus of any kind, selecting only such as can be practiced in the privacy of your own room, without assistance from an instructor or paraphernalia of any kind. Dumb bells, Indian clubs, etc., are valuable after a certain degree of muscular improvement has been attained, but when that point is reached we should advise the individual to join a gymnasium and practice further development under a competent instructor.

All the exercises given have been proved of great value in building up the system, and are designed as aids to the preservation of health and the upbuilding of weakly people--not to develop trained athletes. These exercises bring into play a number of muscles that are not called into general use, and thus promote harmonious development of the whole body.

PART VII.

THE DIET QUESTION.

As we have already stated, the human system is in a state of constant change. Disintegration of tissue is taking place during every moment of existence, and the preservation of health depends upon the prompt elimination of the waste material. But the destruction of tissue, due to the daily friction of life, must be made good, and this replacement of substance is effected by the food we eat. It becomes a matter of vital importance, therefore, to every individual to consider the question of eating from the rational standpoint. Owing to the increased prosperity of recent years and the luxurious mode of living rendered possible by it, people have been betrayed into many reprehensible gastronomic practices. In the olden days, when man toiled hard for existence, food was produced within his own immediate radius and luxuries were unknown; but now, with rapid ocean transportation, the ends of the earth are ransacked and laid under tribute to furnish delicacies to tempt the palate. The ease with which food may now be procured and the almost illimitable variety offered to man for his selection has tempted him into indulgences that have been productive of much evil. Although over indulgence in eating is a very ancient offense, yet, as before stated, the multiplicity of foods has given an impetus to this injurious habit, in combination with the cunningly devised methods of preparation which the modern cook has evolved.

It is a grave mistake to suppose that it is necessary to eat a large quantity of food to become healthy and strong. The system only needs sufficient nourishment to repair the waste that has taken place. Besides, the digestive fluids are not secreted in an indefinite quantity, but in proportion to the immediate need. Hence, food taken in excess of requirements, being only partially digested, acts as a foreign substance; i. e., a poison, and in addition unduly taxes the system to dispose of the unnecessary waste.

Hunger is the natural expression of the needs of the system for nutrition. Appetite is the index as to the quantity of food that should be taken to replace the loss by waste. It should never be overruled. Appetite is a wise provision of Nature. Gluttony is a degrading habit. Yet numbers of people attempt to justify the gratification of their gluttonous proclivities by the statement that they are "blessed with a good appetite," while the truth of the matter is, they are cursed with an inordinate lust for food. If people were more temperate in the pleasures of the table, the purveyors of remedies for dyspepsia would find their incomes considerably lessened. Satisfy your hunger, by all means, but do not pander to the vice of gluttony.

Instead of "eating to live," a large proportion of people simply "live to eat." But sooner or later Nature exacts the penalty for violation of one of her cardinal laws, which is "temperance." An outraged stomach will not always remain quiescent, and when the reaction comes, the offender realizes that "they who sow the wind shall reap the whirlwind."

But people may, and do, continually do violence to that long suffering organ, the stomach, without being gluttons--we refer to the habit, so universally practiced in this country, of bolting the food without properly masticating it. So long as this iniquitous practice is persisted in, and the equally hurtful one of swallowing large quantities of liquids with the meals, and so long as sufficient time is not given the food to digest, just so long will you suffer from a disordered stomach. Speaking generally, Americans are a nation of dyspeptics, because they are perpetually in a hurry. The acquisition of wealth, in moderation, is a commendable pursuit, but it is the height of folly to sacrifice the priceless jewel of health to acquire it. But it is a fact, nevertheless, that the average American considers eating an unprofitable interference with business, without stopping to weigh the advantages of sound health against the almighty dollar.

This habit must be abandoned by those who are addicted to it, before they can expect to regain health or preserve it. Strange, is it not, that a race, proverbial for having an eye to the main chance, should fail to recognize the financial wisdom of husbanding their health, a factor so important in successful business enterprises! They might, with advantage, copy the example of John Bull in the matter of eating.

The average Englishman regards his meals as a solemn responsibility, and tarries long at the table. The consequence is that with them dyspepsia is the exception and not, as with Americans, the rule.

What to eat, when to eat and how to eat are questions more nearly involving the health and happiness of humanity than is generally recognized.

WHAT TO EAT.

From the days of Pythagoras down to the present time it has been a moot question whether a vegetable or meat diet was best for man. Each side can present equally strong arguments; each can point to exceptional instances of physical development under the different methods; each can point to ill results that follow rigid adherence to one method or the other, so that the natural inference would be that a happy mean between the two extremes presents the only rational solution of the question.

Even the most rabid partisan of the meat diet will readily admit that the flesh of animals is not indispensable to existence; while, on the other hand, the fact that the Indians in this country would subsist for months (without apparent discomfort) solely upon a diet of "pemmican" (dried buffalo flesh) affords ample proof that a meat diet is not without its advantages.

Diet is largely a matter of latitude. The whale blubber diet of the Esquimaux would be impossible at the equator, while the fruit and pulse diet of the tropics would prove totally inadequate to support life at the North Pole. Nature always prompts the individual to select the articles of food best adapted to his bodily needs, according to the climatic conditions; hence, when a man endeavors to live on the same dietary in the tropics that he has been accustomed to in the temperate zone, digestive disturbances are sure to follow.

It is one thing to sit at home theorizing about dietetics and settling all the food problems (on paper) to one's entire satisfaction; but it is quite a different matter to practically test the effects of different dietary tables under varying climatic conditions. The writer does not claim to be an expert dietetician, but there are few spots on the habitable globe that he has not visited; scarcely an edible article that he has not partaken of; scarcely a known species of human being that he has not eaten with, except the Patagonians and the Esquimaux; so that he is not entirely without experience, and it may be just possible that practical experience thus gained may be as valuable as statistics compiled in an from data collected from different sources.

We often have the Eastern peoples (notably the Japanese and Hindoos) quoted as examples of physical health and endurance, and the adoption of a vegetarian diet urged on those grounds; but these extremists seem to lose sight of the fact that these peoples are the descendants of vegetarians for centuries past; that they have inherited the tastes of their progenitors, and have evolved their present physical condition through a long period of development along those lines. To say nothing of the impracticability of suddenly converting a nation to the principles of vegetarianism, radical changes abruptly undertaken are always productive of ill effects.

It will help us to a proper understanding of the food question to consider right here what causes old age, or, rather, the physical signs of bodily infirmity that almost invariably accompany it. We are all familiar with the wrinkled body surface, the shrunken limbs and the stiffness of joints that particularly affect the aged, and are so accustomed to regard these outward manifestations of infirmity as inevitable, that few stop to inquire whether it is natural that this should be so. Undoubtedly, these are natural effects, being the result of the operation of natural law, but if mankind lived more in harmony with Nature, these symptoms should not manifest themselves before the age of ninety or a hundred, if even then.

What is termed old age is simply ossification (solidification of the tissues), and this is due to the constant deposition in the system of earthy substances. The result of these deposits being retained in the system is: that there is an excess of mineral matter in the bone tissue, which renders it brittle, and accounts for the susceptibility to fracture in advanced life; it causes a change in the structure of all the blood vessels, great and small, thickening their walls and thus reducing their calibre and also rendering them brittle. With diminished capacity the blood vessels fail to convey the requisite nutrition to the tissues, and a general lowering of the vitality follows. The capillaries no longer supply the skin with its needed pabulum, hence it loses its elasticity and color--grows yellow and forms in furrows. The circulation being sluggish, the deposition of these earthy substances in the neighborhood of the various joints and the muscular structures is facilitated, and we have the stiffness of joints and muscular pains that usually accompany age. The supply of blood to the brain and nerve substance is curtailed in the same manner, and for lack of sustenance these structures commence to decay, which accounts for diminished mental activity and sensory impressions. As the process continues there may be almost complete obliteration of the capillaries, while the larger vessels may become so thickened that their capacity is sometimes reduced three-fifths. Then comes death.

Then, since old age is due to the cause just described, it follows, as a perfectly logical deduction, that if we can prevent the introduction of these substances into the system, or even check them, then the duration of life and preservation of function should be proportionately prolonged.

What are these substances and whence are they obtained? They consist of carbonate and phosphate of lime, principally, with small quantities of the sulphates of lime and magnesia, and a small percentage of other earthy matters. These substances are taken into the system in the food we eat and the water we drink, and it has been estimated that enough lime salts are taken into the system during an average lifetime to form a statue the size of the individual. Of course, the greater part is eliminated by the natural processes, but enough is retained to make ossification a formidable fact. Of the disastrous effects of a preponderance of these mineral salts in the system we have a notable example in the Cretins, a people in the Swiss Alps, who are the victims of premature ossification, their bodies being stunted, rarely attaining a greater height than four feet, and exhibiting all the signs of old age at thirty years; in fact, they seldom live longer than that. In this case the cause is directly traceable to the excess of calcium salts in the drinking water, for although heredity plays an important part in this matter, yet children from other parts, if brought into the region at an early age, soon manifest the symptoms and speedily become Cretins in fact.

Most people are familiar with what is known among housewives as the formation of "fur" in the common tea kettle. This is nothing more nor less than the precipitation of the lime salts by evaporation. Four and five pounds' weight of this substance has been known to collect in this manner in a single vessel in twelve months. Many people are under the mistaken impression that boiling the water removes the lime. Not so. The precipitation only relates to that proportion of the water that has been evaporated; the remainder (in all probability) possesses a slightly higher percentage of solids than it originally did. So great is the proportion of mineral substance taken into the system in drinking water that it is safe to assert that, if after maturity was reached only distilled or other absolutely pure water was partaken of, life would be prolonged fully ten years. Up to the mature age it would be inadvisable, as the salts are necessary for bone formation. Good filtered rain water, or melted snow, are entirely free from mineral deposits, but if they have stood for any length of time it is advisable to boil them before using, to destroy any organic matter.

But it is not in water alone that these pernicious earthy matters are found. All food substances contain them to a greater or lesser extent. The order in which foods stand in the matter of freedom from earthy impurities is as follows: Fruits, fish, animal flesh (including eggs), vegetables, cereals; so that the advocates of a strictly vegetable diet find themselves confronted by the formidable fact that their mainstay is that class of foods that contain the largest proportion of those substances that hasten ossification. Ample proof is at hand that a strictly vegetable diet results in what is known as atheroma (chalky deposit), an affection of the arteries. Dr. Winckler, an enthusiastic food reformer, who wrote extensively on the subject under the nom de plume of Dr. Alanus, and practised a strict vegetarian diet for some years, was compelled to abandon it, on account of the above disease manifesting itself. Numerous similar cases were observed by Raymond, in a monastery of vegetarian friars, and among the poorer Hindoos, who live almost exclusively on rice, this trouble is of frequent occurrence.

The reason of this is obvious. Vegetable food is richer in mineral salts than animal food, and consequently, more are introduced into the blood. There are exceptions, for instance, fruits, which are an ideal food, for several excellent reasons. To commence with, they contain less earthy matter than any other known organic substance; they contain upward of 70 per cent. of the purest kind of distilled water-- distilled in Nature's laboratory; and distilled water is an admirable solvent, and is ready for immediate absorption into the blood, and, lastly, the starch of the fruit has, by the sun's action, been converted into glucose, and is practically ready for assimilation. in order as follows: Dates, figs, bananas, prunes, apples, grapes.

Bread has long been known as the "staff of life," and although it forms the main dietary staple for large numbers of people, that does not in any way prove its eligibility as an article of food. We have seen that cereals contain a very large proportion of inorganic matter (the mineral salts), and wheat is as richly endowed in this respect as any of its fellows. Wheat is rich in heat producing qualities, which is due to the quantity of starch it contains. Now, this starch must be converted into glucose before the system can appropriate it, and as exhaustive experiments have shown that not more than four per cent. of the starch is converted by the ptyalin in the saliva, the principal work of dealing with the starch devolves upon the duodenum, or second stomach, the fluids of the main stomach having no action upon it.

Now, this extra and unnecessary work falling upon the duodenum entails a delay in the process of digestion, and a corresponding delay in assimilation, so a habit of intestinal inactivity is induced, and the seeds of constipation are sown, because the starchy foods, being slow in giving up their nutritive elements, the refuse is proportionately backward in being eliminated. Fruits, on the contrary, although equally rich in heat producing qualities, yet on account of the previous natural transmutation of starch into glucose, are in a condition for immediate appropriation by the system, and consequently absorption of nutrition and elimination of waste are equally prompt. This partially explains the aperient action of fruits, although there is a chemical reason also. For the reasons above stated, lightly baked bread should never be eaten; it should be toasted thoroughly brown first, by which the first step in the conversion of the starch is accomplished.

Regarding the relative digestibility of white and brown (whole wheat) bread there is considerable diversity of opinion, but in a series of experiments described by Dr. John B. Coppock, in the "Herald of Health," England, it was shown that in equal portions of 100 ounces, 1/4 ounce more of the white bread was digested, than of the brown; but the proportion of Proteids (muscle and tissue forming constituents) digested, was as follows: white bread, 85 1/2 ounces; brown bread, 88 3/4 ounces, or 3 1/4 ounces more nutrition obtained from the brown bread than from the white. In any event, we are forced to the conclusion that as an article of food, bread has hitherto had a value placed upon it to which it was not legitimately entitled.

Nature has designed albumen as the staple of nutrition for man, and primarily, vegetable albumen; hence fruits form as nearly as possible a perfect food, containing, as they do, this important constituent in addition to the advantages previously mentioned.

Nuts are an excellent article of diet, as they contain a large percentage of proteid (muscle-forming) substance, and fats--both in a state of almost absolute purity, but are somewhat deficient in starch. To those who feel that they really cannot do without meat, nuts certainly offer the best substitute. There are preparations of nuts on the markets now, called nut-meats, but our advice would be, to eat all nuts without preparation, only being careful to masticate them thoroughly. The peanut is the first in rank for nutritive value, next comes the chestnut, and third, the walnut.

Our objection to nut-meats applies to all forms of concentrated foods, that is, that they do not give the digestive functions the proper amount of exercise. They do not afford sufficient opportunity for mastication, hence the food is not properly insalivated. And, again, in normal conditions, Nature demands a certain amount of bulk, that the digestive organs may have something to contract upon. It is the nature of the muscular structures to grow if exercised, and there is no reason to doubt that the stomach and intestinal muscles respond to this stimulus. Bulk is especially necessary in the intestinal canal, to supply a certain amount of irritative stimulation, for the purpose of exciting peristalsis. That is one reason why whole wheat bread is preferable to white, on account of the bran, which not only supplies the bulk, but favors elimination by its irritative action.

Before proceeding any further we would call attention to the following table, showing the nutritive ingredients in food substances, and their several functions. The ingredients are classified in four divisions: 1, Proteids; 2, Fats;

3, Starches, or carbohydrates; 4, Mineral matters. This is the main classification; but to enable it to be better understood, we subdivide it as follows:

Protein.

a. Albuminoids: e. g. albumen (white of egg); casein (curd) of milk; myosin, the basis of muscle (lean meat); gluten of wheat, etc.

b. Gelatinoids: e. g. collagen of tendons; ossein of bones, which yield gelatin or glue. Meats and fish contain very small quantities of so-called "extractives." They include kreatin and allied compounds, and are the chief ingredients of beef tea and meat extract. They contain nitrogen, and hence are commonly classed with protein.)

Fats.

e. g. fat of meat; fat (butter) of milk; olive oil; oil of corn, wheat, etc.

Carbohydrates.

e. g. sugar, starch, cellulose (woody fibre).

Mineral Matters.

e. g. calcium phosphate or phosphate of lime; sodium chloride (common salt).

In this classification, water is not taken into account, for the reason that it is not a true nutrient, although of vital importance to the body. Now, let us consider what ultimately becomes of these substances--how Nature utilizes them in the physical economy. Protein is used to build up the solid tissues of the body, the muscles and tendons. It is also a source of nutrition for brain and nerve substance, and partially serves as fuel. Fats simply form fatty tissue and serve as fuel to maintain the heat of the body, by combustion or oxidation. Carbohydrates mainly serve as fuel, owing to the large percentage of carbon they contain, which readily unites with the oxygen. The mineral matters, which are also largely obtained from water, are employed in the formation of bone, and are also utilized in the blood and in other ways.

Thus we see that each constituent of the food substance fulfills a specific purpose, and the secret of a correct and nutritious diet lies in the selection of such foods as will furnish the proper proportion of each constituent to serve the purpose for which it is designed. Any deviation from this rule must of necessity result in digestive disturbance, more or less, and although one or two digressions from the path of correct alimentation may not result in anything worse than a slight inconvenience, yet persistence in dietetic errors will inevitably terminate in physical demoralization.

Authorities differ as to the actual proportion the nutritive ingredients should bear to each other in the daily ration; but after comparing the statements advanced by different food experts. We think the following figures will represent a fair average of the various tables. The reader will see that 100 parts of carbo-hydrates is taken as the basis of calculation, the figures opposite the other ingredients representing the proportion they should bear to the basic figure.

Carbo-hydrates (carbonaceous material, starch, sugar, etc.), fat, and heat formers, 100 parts.

Proteids (nitrogenous material) muscle, tissue and brain formers 40 parts.

Fats (animal fats, butter, etc.), fuel formers 32 parts.

Mineral salts, 6 parts.

Water 670 parts.

With the above table in mind, it will be easy to select foods that will furnish, when combined, the proper proportion of each ingredient--that is--approximately, and to assist in the selection, we subjoin a condensed list of the more important articles of food, showing the percentage of each ingredient, as proved by analysis. We would call attention to the fact that animal foods may slightly differ in the ratio of the ingredients, owing to the food upon which the animal has been raised, and its physical condition; and, owing to peculiarities of soil, vegetable foods may differ in like manner, but for practical purposes it will be found sufficiently correct.

IN 100 PARTS.

*Lean Beef Proteids. 20.2 Starches. 0.0 Fats. 3.6 Salts. 2.0

*Fat Proteids. 16.9 Starches. 0.0 Fats. 3.6 Salts. 2.0

*Mutton Proteids. 17.1 Starches. 0.0 Fats. 5.7 Salts. 1.3

*Veal Proteids. 18.8 Starches. 0.0 Fats. 4.4 Salts. 0.5

*Pork Proteids. 14.5 Starches. 0.0 Fats. 37.3 Salts. 0.8

*Poultry Proteids. 21.0 Starches. 0.0 Fats. 3.8 Salts. 1.2

*Smoked Ham Proteids. 24.0 Starches. 0.0 Fats. 36.5 Salts. 10.1

*Mackerel Proteids. 23.5 Starches. 0.0 Fats. 6.7 Salts. 1.0

*Cod Proteids. 27.0 Starches.0.0 Fats.0.3 Salts.22.0

*White of Egg Proteids. 20.4 Starches. 0.0 Fats. 0.0 Salts. 1.6

*Yolk of Egg Proteids. 16.0 Starches. 0.0 Fats. 30.7 Salts. 1.3

*Cow's Milk Proteids. 4.2 Starches. 4.5 Fats. 3.7 Salts. 0.7

*Cheese Proteids. 28.0 Starches. 1.0 Fats. 23.0 Salts. 7.0

*Butter Proteids. 2.0 Starches. 1.0 Fats. 85.0 Salts. 1.0

*Cabbage Proteids. 5.0 Starches. 7.8 Fats. 0.5 Salts. 1.2

*Asparagus Proteids. 1.9 Starches. 2.7 Fats. 0.2 Salts. 0.5

*Mushrooms Proteids. 2.5 Starches. 4.7 Fats. 0.2 Salts. 0.7

*Potatoe Proteids. 2.2 Starches. 21.8 Fats. 0.2 Salts. 1.0

*Sweet Potatoe Proteids. 1.0 Starches. 25.2 Fats. 0.2 Salts. 2.7

*Celery Proteids. 1.5 Starches. 0.8 Fats. 0.4 Salts. 0.8

*French Beans Proteids. 23.7 Starches. 55.6 Fats. 2.2 Salts. 3.7

*Lima Beans Proteids. 21.9 Starches. 60.0 Fats. 1.9 Salts. 2.9

*Green Peas Proteids. 6.3 Starches. 12.0 Fats. 0.5 Salts. 0.8

*Lentils Proteids. 24.8 Starches. 54.7 Fats. 1.8 Salts. 2.4

*Wheat Flour Proteids. 11.6 Starches. 71.0 Fats. 1.3 Salts. 1.6

*Barley Flour Proteids. 10.5 Starches. 66.7 Fats. 2.4 Salts. 2.6

*Oatmeal Proteids. 12.8 Starches. 65.6 Fats. 5.6 Salts. 3.6

*Lentil Flour Proteids. 25.4 Starches. 57.3 Fats. 1.8 Salts. 2.6

*Arrowroot Proteids. 0.8 Starches. 83.5 Fats. 0.0 Salts. 0.3

*Chestnut Proteids. 14.6 Starches. 60.0 Fats. 2.4 Salts. 3.3

*Sweet Almond Proteids. 23.5 Starches. 7.8 Fats. 53.0 Salts. 3.0

*Peanut Proteids. 28.3 Starches. 1.8 Fats. 46.2 Salts. 3.3

*Walnut Proteids. 15.8 Starches. 13.0 Fats. 57.4 Salts. 2.0

*Apple Proteids. 0.4 Starches. 7.2 Fats. 0.0 Salts. 0.5

*Cherry Proteids. 0.7 Starches. 10.2 Fats. 0.0 Salts. 0.7

*Grape Proteids. 0.6 Starches. 14.2 Fats. 0.0 Salts. 0.5

*Banana Proteids. 4.9 Starches. 19.2 Fats. 0.6 Salts. 1.1

*Dates Proteids. 6.6 Starches. 54.0 Fats. 0.2 Salts. 1.6

*Figs Proteids. 6.1 Starches. 60.5 Fats. 0.9 Salts. 2.3

*Honey Proteids. 0.8 Starches. 74.6 Fats. 0.9 Salts. 0.2

TABLE A.

Showing the relative digestibility of various foods.

* Beef, round

PROTEIN. Digestible. 23.0 Undigestible. 0.0

FATS. Digestible. 8.1 Undigestible. 0.9

CARBOHYDRATES. Digestible. 0.0 Undigestible. 0.0

MINERAL MATERS. 1.3

WATER. 66.7

* Beef, sirloin

PROTEIN. Digestible. 20.0 Undigestible. 0.0

FATS. Digestible. 17.1 Undigestible. 1.9

CARBOHYDRATES. Digestible. 0.0 Undigestible. 0.0

MINERAL MATERS. 1.0

WATER. 60.0

*Pork, very fat.

PROTEIN. Digestible. 3.0 Undigestible. 0.0

FATS. Digestible. 74.5 Undigestible. 6.0

CARBOHYDRATES. Digestible. - Undigestible. -

MINERAL MATERS. 6.5

WATER. 10.0

*Haddock.

PROTEIN. Digestible. 17.1 Undigestible. 0.0

FATS. Digestible. 0.3 Undigestible. -

CARBOHYDRATES. Digestible. 0.0 Undigestible. 0.0

MINERAL MATERS. 1.2

WATER. 81.4

*Mackerel

PROTEIN. Digestible. 18.8 Undigestible. 0.0

FATS. Digestible. 7.4 Undigestible. 0.8

CARBOHYDRATES. Digestible. 0.0 Undigestible. 0.0

MINERAL MATERS. 1.4

WATER. 71.6

*Hen's eggs

PROTEIN. Digestible. 13.4 Undigestible. 0.0

FATS. Digestible. 9.4 Undigestible. 2.4

CARBOHYDRATES. Digestible. 0.7 Undigestible. 0.0

MINERAL MATERS. 1.0

WATER. 73.1

*Cow's Milk

PROTEIN. Digestible. 3.4 Undigestible. 0.0

FATS. Digestible. 3.6 Undigestible. 0.1

CARBOHYDRATES. Digestible. 4.8 Undigestible. 0.0

MINERAL MATERS. 0.7

WATER. 87.4

*Cheese, whole milk

PROTEIN. Digestible. 27.1 Undigestible. 0.0

FATS. Digestible. 34.6 Undigestible. 0.9

CARBOHYDRATES. Digestible. 2.3 Undigestible. 0.0

MINERAL MATERS. 3.9

WATER. 31.2

*Butter

PROTEIN. Digestible. 1.0 Undigestible. -

FATS. Digestible. 85.8 Undigestible. 1.7

CARBOHYDRATES. Digestible. 0.5 Undigestible. -

MINERAL MATERS. 2.0

WATER. 9.0

*Oleomargarine

PROTEIN. Digestible. 0.4 Undigestible. -

FATS. Digestible. 83.9 Undigestible. 3.3

CARBOHYDRATES. Digestible. 0.0 Undigestible. -

MINERAL MATERS. 2.1

WATER. 10.3

*Sugar

PROTEIN. Digestible. 0.3 Undigestible. -

FATS. Digestible. - Undigestible. -

CARBOHYDRATES. Digestible. 96.7 Undigestible. 0.0

MINERAL MATERS. 0.8

WATER. 2.2

*Wheat flour (very fine).

PROTEIN. Digestible. 7.6 Undigestible. 1.3

FATS. Digestible. 1.0 Undigestible. -

CARBOHYDRATES. Digestible. 74.4 Undigestible. 0.8

MINERAL MATERS. 0.3

WATER. 14.6

* Wheat flour (Medium)

PROTEIN. Digestible. 9.5 Undigestible. 2.1

FATS. Digestible. 0.8 Undigestible. -

CARBOHYDRATES. Digestible. 70.4 Undigestible. 1.8

MINERAL MATERS. 0.4

WATER. 15.0

*Wheat flour (coarse whole wheat)

PROTEIN. Digestible. 8.2 Undigestible. 2.7

FATS. Digestible. 1.8 Undigestible. -

CARBOHYDRATES. Digestible. 66.4 Undigestible. 5.3

MINERAL MATERS. 1.2

WATER. 14.4

* Wheat Bread.

PROTEIN. Digestible. 7.7 Undigestible. 1.2

FATS. Digestible. 1.9 Undigestible. -

CARBOHYDRATES. Digestible. 54.9 Undigestible. 0.6

MINERAL MATERS. 1.0

WATER. 32.7

*Black bread.

PROTEIN. Digestible. 4.5 Undigestible. 1.6

FATS. Digestible. 1.8 Undigestible. -

CARBOHYDRATES. Digestible. 43.3 Undigestible. 5.3

MINERAL MATERS. 1.5

WATER. 43.8

*peas.

PROTEIN. Digestible. 19.7 Undigestible. 3.2

FATS. Digestible. - Undigestible. -

CARBOHYDRATES. Digestible. 55.7 Undigestible. 2.1

MINERAL MATERS. 2.5

WATER. 15.0

*Corn (maize) Meal.

PROTEIN. Digestible. 7.9 Undigestible. 1.2

FATS. Digestible. 3.8 Undigestible. -

CARBOHYDRATES. Digestible. 68.7 Undigestible. 2.3

MINERAL MATERS. 1.6

WATER. 14.5

*Rice.

PROTEIN. Digestible. 6.2 Undigestible. 1.2

FATS. Digestible. 0.4 Undigestible. -

CARBOHYDRATES. Digestible. 78.7 Undigestible. 0.7

MINERAL MATERS. 0.4

WATER. 12.4

*Potatoes.

PROTEIN. Digestible. 1.5 Undigestible. 0.5

FATS. Digestible. 0.2 Undigestible. -

CARBOHYDRATES. Digestible. 19.7 Undigestible. 1.6

MINERAL MATERS. 1.0

WATER. 75.5

*Turnips.

PROTEIN. Digestible. 0.7 Undigestible. 0.3

FATS. Digestible. 0.2 Undigestible. -

CARBOHYDRATES. Digestible. 5.6 Undigestible. 1.3

MINERAL MATERS. 0.7

WATER. 91.2

Since the elements are seldom, if ever, found in the proper proportion in any food substances, it becomes necessary to exercise judgement in selecting them, so that something like a well balanced diet may be obtained; so as a further aid to enable the reader to make his selection judiciously, we would call attention to Table A and Table B below. Table A shows the proportion of various foods that is ordinarily digested, while Table B points out the time required for different articles of food to digest.

TABLE B.

LENGTH OF TIME REQUIRED FOR DIGESTION OF DIFFERENT ARTICLES OF FOOD.

Hours.

Apples, raw, 2:00 Barley, boiled, 2:00 Beef, roasted, 3:00 Beefsteak, broiled, 3:00 Beef, broiled, 4:00 Beets, boiled, 3:45 Brains, animal, boiled, 1:45 Bread, corn, baked, 3:15 Bread, wheat, baked, 3:30 Butter, melted, 3:30 Cabbage, raw, 2:30 Cabbage, with vinegar, 2:00 Cabbage, boiled, 4:30 Cake, corn, baked, 3:00 Cake, sponge, baked, 2:30 Catfish, fried, 3:30 Cheese, old strong, 3:30 Chicken, fricasseed, 2:45 Corn and beans, boiled, 3:45 Custard, baked, 2:45 Duck, roasted, 4:00 Dumpling, apple, boiled, 3: 00 Eggs, hard boiled, 3:30 Eggs, soft boiled, 3:00 Eggs, fried, 3:30 Eggs, roasted, 2:15 Eggs, raw, 2:00 Fowls, boiled, 4: 00 Fowls, roasted, 4: 00 Goose, roasted, 2: 30 Lamb, boiled, 2: 30 Milk, boiled, 2: 00 Milk, raw, 2: 15 Mutton, roasted, 3:15 Mutton, broiled, 3:00 Mutton, boiled, 3:00 Oysters, raw, 2:55 Oysters, roasted, 3:15 Oysters, stewed, 3:30 Pig, roasted, 2:30 Pigs' feet, soused, 1:00 Pork, roasted, 5:15 Pork, salted and fried, 4:15 Potatoes, Irish, boiled, 3:30 Potatoes, Irish, roasted, 2:30 Rice, boiled, 1:00 Salmon, salted, 4:00 Soup, barley, boiled, 1:30 Soup, bean, 3:30 Soup, chicken, 3:00 Soup, mutton, 3:30 Soup, oyster, 3:30 Tapioca, boiled, 2:00 Tripe, soused, 1:00 Trout, salmon, boiled, 1:30 Trout, salmon, fried, 1:30 Turkey, roast, 2:30 Turkey, boiled, 2:30 Turnips, boiled, 3:30 Veal, broiled, 4:00 Veal, fried, 4:30 Vegetables and meat hashed, 2:30 Venison steak, 1:35

We have seen that certain elements are necessary in our food for the proper replenishment of the waste that is perpetually going on, and that they must be combined in proper proportions, so that no one part of the body shall be over-nourished at the expense of the others--no organ overtaxed, but that all may be harmoniously developed.

Opinions may, and do, differ as to the source from which this sustenance for the body should be obtained whether from the animal or vegetable kingdoms, or both, and while admitting that vegetarianism and flesh-eating both have their advantages and disadvantages, our own conscientious conviction is, that the true solution of the question is to be found in the happy medium--that a mixed diet is the best for mankind under existing conditions.

The main argument of our vegetarian friends against the practice of flesh-eating is the humanitarian one. We are familiar with all the objections urged--the brutalizing effect upon the human mind of so much ruthless bloodshed--of the sacredness of life, and of man's presumption in daring to deprive a living creature of existence; but with all due respect to the sensibilities of these worthy people, we are inclined to think that the argument is scarcely tenable. We do not wish to be understood as defending the cruelties that are said to be practised in the abattoirs; but the taking of life is inseparable from existence. It is simply a question of degree. There is a sect in India, the members of which are so scrupulous regarding the sanctity of life that they carefully brush every step of the path in front of them, lest they should inadvertently step upon any creeping thing. In this, they lift the burden of responsibility from themselves for any wanton injury; but the microscope has shown us that there is a countless world of infinitesimal life all around us, and that it is practically impossible to draw a breath, or drink a mouthful of water, without destroying some living thing. If we accept the teaching of the Scriptures, that not a sparrow falls to the ground without the knowledge of the Creator, then we must conclude that the life of the ant is of as much importance in His eyes as that of the ox or sheep. We repeat, we are not posing as advocates of indiscriminate and wanton slaughter, but on utilitarian grounds, we consider the use of the flesh of animals, as a food, justifiable.

If we needed any scriptural authority for the practice, we could point to the Hebrews, who (according to Holy Writ) received through Moses not only permission to use meat as an article of diet, but instructions for the killing of the selected animals, together with injunctions to avoid the flesh of certain kinds; and they may be cited as a striking example of the value of a mixed diet.

Here we have one of the most ancient races of the earth--a race that has endured the most terrible persecutions that ever befell a people, yet have survived it all, and are to-day a robust and unusually prolific race; while intellectually and morally they are surpassed by none. They are a greater power in the world than any other race, by reason of their finance and business instincts. There is no question but that the sanitary system of living established by Moses has been the principle factor in perpetuating this hardy race; and a mixed diet was and is an integral part of that system. It may also be confidently claimed that the teachings of the Bible, along these lines, have been in a large degree responsible for the position occupied by the Christian nations in the world to-day.

However, we have no desire to impose our views upon our readers, and having given expression to our sentiments, we return to the main question.

Having disposed of the question, "what to eat," we will consider another matter, almost equally important, and that is:

How To Eat.

The one fundamental principle underlying this question is thorough mastication, and we cannot too strongly impress upon our readers the necessity for its proper observance. We have already stated that digestion cornmences in the mouth--that by the action of the saliva, the starchy matter in food is converted into glucose. It is therefore necessary that the saliva should be brought into intimate contact with every part of the bolus; and for that purpose thorough mastication is absolutely necessary. In addition, the separation of the food into small fragments, by the teeth, assists stomach digestion, by permitting the gastric juice freer access to the food. It is stated that Mr. Gladstone formed the habit of thorough mastication by making it a rule to count thirty two while masticating each mouthful. Mastication need not be slow to be thorough, although there is an impression to that effect, for, as a matter of fact, quick and vigorous chewing excites the salivary glands to more energetic action.

Drinking at meals should be avoided as much as possible, and whenever any digestive trouble is present, not only should no liquids accompany the meal, but nothing in the form of fluids should be partaken of within half an hour preceding or following a meal, The philosophy of this is apparent, when we reflect that all digestive disturbances are accompanied by imperfect secretion of the gastric juices, and to dilute them with an excess of fluid is to weaken its power of action on the food. It is as if a man, when attempting to dissolve a piece of metal in a powerful acid, should deliberately add water to the acid, and thereby arrest, wholly or in part, the process of decomposition. It is plain, therefore, that although the practice of drinking at meals may help the food to pass more easily down the aesophagus, yet it must inevitably retard digestion when it reaches the stomach.

But the most pernicious practice of all is that of drinking ice water at meals, since, in addition to the ill effects described above, it temporarily paralyzes the stomach-driving the blood away from that organ when it is needed most of all. A fact which should not be lost sight of is, that no physical operation, however slight, can be accomplished without the expenditure of force (nervous energy), even though it be only the winking of an eyelid; and the labor entailed upon the system, of raising the temperature of the stomach to normal figures, after deluging it with ice water, involves a ruinous waste of vital force, in addition to the other reasons urged against it. It cannot be doubted that this essentially American habit is responsible for a large proportion of the dyspepsia that sits like an incubus upon the nation. Every substance taken into the stomach, whether fluid or solid, should be about the same temperature as the body, to be in harmony with natural principles.

All condiments promote indigestion. They over stimulate the stomach, exciting the secreting glands to abnormal action, and irritating the sensitive mucous surface. In addition, they overheat the blood, excite the nervous system, inflame the passions, and are largely responsible for many of the excesses into which men plunge under this unnatural stimulation.

WHEN TO EAT

Is a question that has excited a great deal of discussion of late years. The publication of Dr. Dewey's book, extolling the no-breakfast plan, caused the subject to be debated, with considerable fervor for a time, but the matter remains practically where it was. It is impossible to lay down a hard and fast rule that shall govern all cases, a fact that most theorists seem to lose sight of--hence the collapse of so many promising and alluring schemes. For people in health, we strongly advise the three meals a day system, which experience has shown to be successful. They should be moderate in quantity, and should be eaten as follows: The first, from half an hour to an hour after rising (having previously bathed and exercised); the second, not less than four hours afterwards; the third, not less than five hours later.

This gives the stomach time to rid itself of one meal before the next is introduced, otherwise the undigested food remaining in the stomach prevents that organ from acting properly on the fresh food. It is for this reason that it is unwise to eat between meals, as, when the stomach is occupied by articles of food in various stages of digestion, undigested portions will pass out with the digested food; not only entailing a serious loss of energy and nutrition, but irritating the intestinal canal and creating unnecessary waste to be eliminated.

The above rules, as stated, apply to people in ordinarily good health. In wasting disease it may be necessary to supply nutrition even as often as every half hour; and in all serious digestive troubles it is wiser to eat six times a day than three, the meals to be light, nutritious in quality, and small in quantity, so as not to impose too great a burden at one time on the weakened digestive apparatus.

We will now consider the action of several substances, in common use, that are inimical to health, and that have an especially demoralizing effect upon digestion.

The first of these is alcohol, which only serves as fuel, but does not form tissue. Its best friends in the medical profession no longer claim anything for it but a stimulating effect. Its action on the digestive organs (especially the stomach) is disastrous in the extreme. It destroys the appetite, although it temporarily sustains vigor by unnatural excitation.

Without going so far as to say that a man is lost to all sense of decency because he takes an occasional drink, we will say that it is in nowise necessary to the system--that the habit, indulged in to excess, is the most fatal that can be contracted, and that inasmuch as the majority of people have not sufficient will-power to curb their appetites, the wisest plan is to avoid the use of alcoholic beverages altogether.

The man who is addicted to the excessive use of alcoholic stimulants is overtaxing the vital organs of his body in the most outrageous manner, and although Nature incessantly enters protest against being overworked, he either ignorantly fails to recognize the warnings, or wantonly disregards them. Let us for a few moments consider the work which the heart is called upon to do, and the amount of extra labor imposed upon it by the unwise use of alcohol. The average life of a man is thirty-eight years, and, in a healthy man, the number of heart- beats per minute is seventy, or during an average life, 76,536,740,000. Now, the use of alcohol in anything like an excessive quantity increases the action of the heart ten beats per minute, making 600 extra beats per hour, 14,400 per day, 482,000 per month, 9,784,000 per year, 195,568,000 in twenty years, and 372,793,000 in a lifetime of thirty-eight years. Or, supposing a man should live fifty years, the number of pulsations of the heart during that period, at the normal rate, would be 917, 239,680. Now, if ten extra beats be added to this, for, say the last twenty-five years, we find that the heart is called upon to make 91,840,000 extra beats. Think of that enormous amount of additional work imposed upon a delicate, complex piece of mechanism like the human heart!

But that is not the worst of it. The heart should rest and sleep when we do. During sleep, the character of the beats is different from what it is during our waking hours--the beats are made singly and deliberately, with a pause between, for the heart is taking its necessary rest, to fit it for its functions on the morrow; but, if we take alcohol into the system before retiring, then the heart works harder during sleep than a healthy man's when he is awake.

Is it any wonder that we hear of so many cases of heart failure? Is it strange that the average duration of human life is steadily and surely growing shorter? Three-score and ten was the average number of years for man to sojourn here, it is now thirty-eight, and will inevitably become still less someday if man persists in wilfully violating the laws that govern his being.

Tea and coffee are substances which neither form tissue nor serve as fuel, and may be banished from the table with decided advantage. Few people realize that the difference between the drinking of alcohol and tea is simply a question of degree. It is true that the consequences of excessive tea drinking are not as severe as those from over-indulgence in ardent spirits, but the pernicious effects of the constant drinking of strong infusions of tea justify us in calling the practice a serious menace to health. Tea leaves contain from 2 to 4 per cent. of caffeine, or theme, which is an alkaloid, and always found in combination with tannin. They also contain a volatile oil, which is the source of the aroma, and in addition possess a sedative quality. Tannin is a powerful astringent, and hence is strongly provocative of constipation. Its action upon the mucous surface of the stomach is highly detrimental to that organ, as it arrests the excretion of the gastric juice by its contractile effect upon the glands. Its constant use will almost invariably result in digestive disturbances, and will certainly aggravate such troubles, if previously existing. It is true that a cup of hot tea is a refreshing beverage, but not more so than a cup of hot milk--in fact, it is the heat that imparts the sense of comfort experienced on drinking it. Children should never be allowed to drink either tea or coffee, as the seeds of a baneful habit may be sown, for in tea, as in dram drinking, it is a habit easily acquired.

The above remarks apply in a less degree to the frequent use of coffee. The constant use of these substances produce the following results--first, increase of circulation, rise in pulse, a desire to frequently pass urine, and an exhilaration resembling intoxication. Tea tasters, as is well known, are subject to headache and giddiness, and prone to attacks of paralysis. The votaries of the tea and coffee cup by far outnumber those of Bacchus, so that granting that the drinking of these beverages is a little less severe in its constitutional effects, yet the greater prevalence of the habit renders them equal to alcohol in their destructive effects.

GENERAL SUGGESTIONS.

One of the causes that conduce to digestive disturbances is that of solitary eating. Owing to the strenuousness of modern city life, many people, of both sexes, are compelled to practice the most rigid economy, which, in a large proportion of cases, involves what is known as "light housekeeping," or preparing a part, if not all of their meals over a gas jet in their room. In the case of the male housekeeper, this generally means that when he seats himself to eat he places his book or paper in front of him, to beguile the time; the consequence being that he not only calls the blood away from the stomach, where it is needed, but, engrossed in his reading, he masticates imperfectly, or suddenly coming to himself, he finds that he has been so intent on his reading that his food has become cold, whereupon he devours it in haste. Women are not such great sinners in this respect as men; but are equally culpable in another direction. It is a pretty well-known fact that a woman would just as soon not eat at all as to eat alone, and as a result frequently deprives herself of the necessary amount of nutrition. In fact, she impairs her digestion by not giving it sufficient work to do, while the man ruins his by spasmodically overtaxing it. For the above reasons, the boarding house (much as it leaves to be desired) is preferable as an abiding place for hundreds of men and women who are too busy by day and too tired at night to pay proper attention to the physical needs of the system. Companionship at meals is a most desirable thing, especially if it is congenial, and light, cheerful conversation, with a little hilarity intermingled, is an excellent aid to digestion.

This is, no doubt, due to mental influence. The whole of the alimentary process is under the control of the nervous system, which has its seat in the brain, consequently, a cheerful mental attitude favors digestion. It is well known that a fit of anger may temporarily stop digestion. The mind exerts such a vast influence over every function that it is impossible to set bounds to it. We are the creatures of habit. We eat so many times a day, from sheer force of habit. We habituate ourselves to partake of articles of food against which, at first, the senses rebel, by the same force; but it is left wholly to mans reasoning powers whether his habits shall be cultivated according to the needs of the system. If they are, perfect nutrition will be established; if they are not, he is worse off than the animal who knows only to follow the instincts of the original habits of the species. A man can exercise his will power to partake of a diet which his taste had not been able to appreciate, yet no will power can ever provide good nutrition out of a diet against which taste constantly rebels. Consciousness of the digestive organs is an offense to them. The more a man is conscious of his stomach, the less will be its capacity for performing good service; therefore, a dyspeptic should never attempt to follow a course of experimental dietetics with himself, for if he watches his stomach after his carefully selected meal, to see how it will serve him, he will always find abnormal symptoms. It is never wise to expect anything but good results from anything which has been allowed to pass beyond the palate, for that is Nature's infallible safeguard, its province being to reject every objectionable thing.

We would again remind the reader that one of the most important offices of the lungs is to promote the movement of the blood and lymph currents throughout the body. Active respiration assists all forms of lymph absorption, but gives special aid to the absorption of food substances from the stomach and intestines, because these particular lymph vessels are situated so close to the chest cavity that they are more directly under the influence of the suction action of the chest.

A few minutes spent in vigorous deep breathing exercise after each meal is one of the best means of remedying the sense of heaviness and weight of which so many complain after eating.

Thus we see that deep breathing, by favoring absorption, promotes the nourishment of the body will assist in building tissue, in fact. Oxygen is a vital necessity for the body, and it is necessary to absorb a large quantity for the actual needs of the system, while all absorbed over the quantity means added nutrition. Now, deep, or diaphragmatic breathing, infallibly increases the lung capacity, so that the possibility for absorption of oxygen is increased, and health and strength promoted. Deep breathing is as necessary for the proper absorption and assimilation of nutrition as the selection of a well-balanced diet. It has saved thousands of lives, and is a factor in promoting health that cannot be disregarded.

"Order is Heaven's first law," and nowhere is this law better exemplified than in the human body. Order, or regularity, is an essential for success in human affairs--moral, mental, or physical; but especially in the latter. The successful conduct of large business organizations is only possible by regularity in the performance of every detail of duty.

If this be so when only physical results are involved, how much more so is it where vital interests are at stake? The human body is a wonderfully complex piece of mechanism, and if left to itself or rather to natural guidance, its manifold functions are performed with unfailing regularity; and regularity in function means health-- irregularity, disease.

Mark the rhythmic regularity of respiration, or of the heart's contractions! Long continued regularity begets habit, which is a form of automatism; hence the necessity of regularity in action along fixed lines, and in consonance with physiological law, that good habits only may be formed.

Good habits are absolutely essential to health, which is equivalent to saying that regularity in living is an imperative necessity to that end. Regularity in rising and retiring; regularity in eating and drinking; regularity in exercise, all are equally important.

Not only does this regularity of conduct conduce to the attainment and maintenance of perfect health, but it enables the individual to accomplish more within the limits of the day, partly by economizing time, and partly by the added vigor due to improved health.

First, regularity in the hours of rising and retiring, namely, regulating the minimum period to be devoted to sleep. There is much conflict of opinion as to the amount of sleep necessary for the average adult. We have in mind an old saying which runs as follows: "Six hours' sleep for a man, seven for a woman, and eight for a fool." This is somewhat arbitrary, and, moreover, is not in harmony with physiological law. In the first place, no hard and fast rule can be laid down that will cover all cases. Apart from the difference of sex, there are temperamental conditions which vary with every case. We are decidedly of the opinion that eight hours' sleep is necessary for the adult individual. It has been affirmed by some authorities that the more the individual sleeps the longer he will live, which is a perfectly rational claim, in view of the fact that night is Nature's repair time, when she is busy at work replacing the ravages committed by wear and tear during the day. It is a well known fact that nearly all growth takes place during sleep.

Again, it is a fact not generally known that the heart receives no nourishment during the period of contraction, owing to the pressure upon the arteries which supply it with nutriment. It is only during the infinitesimal pause between the contractions that these arteries can carry blood to the heart tissue; hence during sleep the heart- beats differ from those of our waking hours, being fewer in number, and with a more decided pause between. Now, the heart being to the body what the mainspring is to a watch, the necessity of affording it ample time for recuperation becomes apparent.

Having stated that eight hours' sleep is the minimum amount for the individual, the question of regularity presents itself, and this should be understood to refer especially to the time of rising, which, unless the individual is in ill health, should be at 6 A. M. This not only proves invaluable in economizing time, but paves the way for regularity in eating, which we will now consider.

There is much diversity of opinion as to the number of meals that should be eaten during the day, and recently the practice of eating only two meals a day has largely obtained. This, although preferable to the practice of eating four and five meals a day, or of indiscriminate lunching between meals, is yet (we consider) running into the other extreme. Unless an exceedingly hearty breakfast is eaten, the tax upon the vitality before the next meal hour arrives is too severe. Our rule, which we commend to our readers, is as follows: Rise at six, then take your bath, either plunge or sponge bath, followed by ten to fifteen minutes of moderate exercise. This, we will say, occupies until seven; then eat a light meal of juicy fruit, such as oranges, grapes or berries, followed by the perusal of the morning newspaper, or, if you are a student, devote an hour to study. At eight o'clock take your proper breakfast, which should consist of some preparation of wheat (with milk or fruit juice), followed by toast, boiled or poached eggs, and a glass of milk. Take a light lunch at 1 P. M., and a moderately good dinner at 7 P. M.

If regularity in the hours for meals be strictly observed, and the quantity and character of the meals carefully considered, the system will rapidly acquire the habit of expecting sustenance at those hours, and regularity, like virtue, will be its own reward.

Next comes the question of exercise. Too little attention is paid to this matter, more especially by those engaged in sedentary occupations; yet it is in the highest degree important that the balance between the mental and physical energies should be maintained. To preserve this balance while the mind is active and the body untaxed, artificial exercise must be practiced, for physical strength cannot be promoted without some kind of bodily exercise. Unused muscles soon become flabby, as athletes and their trainers well know. The best time for taking exercise is, as stated above, just after the morning bath, and it is astonishing what results can be obtained from fifteen minutes of intelligently directed exercise each morning. Here, again, regularity will work wonders. It may be a week or two before you will notice any marked improvement in the muscular condition, but you will be amply repaid by the glow of health which pervades the system as the result of stimulated circulation.

Last, but by no means least, comes the matter of solicitation of the bowels. In this case regularity in solicitation will invariably produce regularity in movement The bowels should be solicited every morning, soon after rising, and every night just before retiring. We only wish that we could impress every one of our readers with the importance of this practice, and of the immense benefit of regularity in the pursuance of it. Just as the stomach acquires the habit of expecting food when regularly supplied to it at stated intervals, even so will the bowels respond to solicitation if regularity be persisted in.

Nature is inexorably opposed to caprice. She executes all her processes in an orderly manner, and if not interfered with, with the greatest regularity, and if man will only co-operate with her by strict regularity in the important duties previously mentioned, the result will be a surprise to him in the form of renewed health and vigor. He will have an unclouded mind, and be ready to face the trials of everyday existence with a courage that nothing can daunt.

But Nature demands an accurate accounting. Man thinks but little of the drafts he is continually making upon his vitality, but sooner or later the account will be presented, and payment exacted in full. There is no such thing as vicarious payment. The debtor must pay in person, and it therefore behooves every man to watch the debit side of his life's ledger, and make a daily balance of his account with Nature.

PART VIII.

TREATMENT OF DISEASE.

HEART DISEASE.

There are numerous affections of the heart, divided into two classes--organic and functional, the former being the more serious; but it is safe to say that seventy-five per cent. of cases belong in the latter class. The most common, and at the same time most serious, of the organic troubles, are pericarditis (inflammation of the heart- envelope), and valvular insufficiency (imperfect closure of the valves). The functional disturbances are (almost without exception) due to digestive difficulties. In the first class, if the case is well advanced and the patient past the meridian of life, recovery is improbable, although life may be considerably prolonged. The second class of cases can be cured, with reasonable certainty, by removing the cause.

TREATMENT.

In pericarditis--the symptoms of which are fever and sharp pain under left nipple, radiating to the armpit, use the "Cascade" daily while the condition is acute; the wet sheet should also be employed daily, the temperature varying with the degree of fever. It is usually the sequel of rheumatism. In valvular insufficiency, which is caused by deposits upon the valves of the heart, the symptoms of which are principally difficulty of respiration, not much pain, but a feeling of uneasiness in the heart region, and a peculiar sound termed "the murmer," to be detected by the stethoscope, the use of the "Cascade" will sometimes effect wonders. It arrests all further deposition of impurities in the blood, thus preventing any further accumulation on the valves, while the increased liquidity and purity of the blood enables it to re-absorb the existing deposits and thus restore normal action. Functional difficulties, as stated, chiefly result from digestive troubles, due to fermentation of food in the stomach and the consequent formation of gas, which frequently collects in large quantities, and by actual pressure impedes the heart's action. The chief symptoms are shortness of breath, palpitation, and great irregularity of the heart's action; sometimes the heart appears to miss a beat altogether. In such cases, a faithful observance of the formula of treatment for dyspepsia (see index) will accomplish surprising results.

ANEMIA.

This is a disease of the blood, characterized by a deficiency of albumen and red corpuscles. It is a disease that more frequently affects women than men; the very young and the very old are most subject to it, and especially, if of a nervous, irritable or hysterical disposition Among the exciting causes are defective hygiene, poor diet, want of, or excessive exercise, grief, or other strong emotions. The symptoms are great pallor, muscular weakness frequent pulse, dizziness, breathlessness on slight exertion and fainting. There is another form of this trouble, known as Essential Anaemia, or Progressive Pernicious Anaemia, which almost invariably terminates in death; while in the first form, or simple anaemia, there is no reason whatever for a fatal result, if treated judiciously.

TREATMENT.

The condition of the blood must be improved, and as the blood is only formed from the food that is eaten, the importance of getting the digestive function into good working order is apparent. Also to supply those elements to the system that the condition of the blood shows to be necessary, all of which can be furnished in properly selected articles of food. The body must be cleansed internally, by means of the "Cascade," using it as frequently as the condition of the patient will permit, without unduly taxing the system. The skin should be kept active by frequent warm or tepid baths, followed by gentle friction with a soft towel. A half pint of hot water should be slowly sipped soon after rising, and no nourishment partaken of for at least half an hour. Gentle exercise should be employed, to promote circulation; or if too weak, substitute massage. Eggs and milk should be freely partaken of. The eggs are preferable raw, beaten in milk, if not, then lightly boiled or poached. Milk should only be taken in quantities of from two to four ounces at a time. Some good preparation of whole wheat should be partaken of once daily for the benefit of the phosphates contained in it, but iron is the element most, needed, and this is to be obtained in the following articles: first and foremost, spinach, then beets, tomatoes, dark skinned grapes and ditto plums. Lastly, and most important, is the practice of deep breathing to thoroughly oxygenate the blood.

BLOOD POISONING.

This may arise from various causes, such as the infection of a wound, contact with some irritating vegetable substance like the poison ivy, or by inhaling noxious gases, or handling certain metals, such as copper and lead; but the most common cause is the re-absorption into the blood, through the intestinal walls, of the waste products of the system; in fact, it may be confidently asserted that ninety-nine per cent. of such cases are due to this cause. When it is considered that a virulent poison introduced in the rectum has been known to cause death in a rabbit within two minutes, the absorptive character of the walls of the colon may be faintly estimated. True, the toxic substances generated in the body are not so rapid in their action, but they are none the less deadly. It is to this that all skin diseases, together with rheumatism, gout, neuralgia and a host of other troubles, are undoubtedly due.

TREATMENT.

Clean out the human cesspool by frequent use of the "Cascade," thus preventing any further deposition of these impure substances in the blood, and keep it clean by more or less constant use. In acute cases, take frequent Turkish baths, to help elimination by way of the skin, and keep that organ active by frequent warm baths and vigorous friction with a moderately coarse towel. Let the diet be plain and moderate, never eating to excess, and drink freely of water, to keep the blood liquid, and practice the habit of breathing deeply, to oxygenate the blood.

CONSUMPTION.

Of all diseases, consumption is the most widespread and destructive to human life. Over 3,000,000 people die annually from this disease. It is not only an acquired disease, but surely preventable, and in its early stages, curable. In the majority of cases it commences just beneath the collar bone, because here is the part of the lung that is least used, the reserve portion, not much used in ordinary breathing. In most of the avocations of life the shoulders are drawn forward, thus cramping the lungs, and weakening them, then the consumption bacillus finds lodgment. A person with healthy lungs might inhale millions of tubercle bacilli daily with impunity, hence the inference is plain--to prevent consumption, distend the lungs fully, by deep breathing, hundreds of times daily.

TREATMENT.

The first thing to be done (if it is in your power) is to go to some quiet country place where you can be sure of the three following essentials--a dry location, pure air, and a plentiful supply of fresh, rich milk. There is an almost universal consensus of opinion now that the open air treatment is of the greatest benefit; therefore, live as much as possible out of doors and sleep with the doors and windows of your room wide open. Never mind, if you have to pile on bed clothing to keep warm--the prime essential is unlimited fresh air. You will soon get used to it, and you are playing for a big stake--

health. If it is impossible to go to the country, then carry out this treatment as closely as possible at your home. It is absolutely necessary to improve the nutrition of the body, that is, to stimulate the digestion and absorbent functions of the stomach and intestines, therefore dispense with all so-called cough medicines. The drugs used to stop a cough are invariably sedatives. Now, no sedative or nauseant is known that does not lock up the natural secretions, and thus lessen the digestive powers. Flushing the colon with the "Cascade" is the first step to improve nutrition. This unlocks the secretions and prepares the stomach for food.

Next, flush the stomach. Then give the stomach food that the organs can digest and assimilate.

For this purpose nothing equals good, rich, fresh milk. Live on milk exclusively for a month at least, taking a tumbler full every half hour--the object being to supply the body with food easily digested, quickly absorbed, and highly nourishing; yet at the same time, in small quantities, that will not overtax the stomach. You will quickly gain in weight, and after a month or two you may commence on solid foods partly, choosing such articles as the Salisbury steak (see treatment for obesity), pure cod liver oil, sweet cream, eggs, toasted whole wheat bread, etc. Ten drops of beechwood creosote morning and night, on a fifty cent respirator, is all the drug treatment necessary, or useful. An external bath for those able to walk about, and a "sponge off" for those confined to bed, must not be neglected. The skin exudes more matter and is more likely .to become clogged in disease than in health. Practise deep breathing assiduously. Improved nutrition is your salvation, and that must come through exercise, diet and fresh air. Spend all the time possible in the open air and in the sun's rays whenever practicable, and pay special attention to the use of the "Cascade." Remember, the cure is in your own hands--depends upon your own courage and perseverance.

CATARRH.

This is a disease resulting from cold. It is the exception rather than the rule, to meet with individuals in our Northern climate who are not afflicted with it in some form or other. It is easier to prevent than cure. Strong, well developed lungs, a clean colon and skin, and catarrh, are seldom found together in the same body. Perfect lung development and a clean colon will alone effect a permanent cure. Keep the feet warm and dry, never go into a hot room and sit or lie, but sleep in a cool, dry atmosphere. The disease takes two different forms, nasal and throat. Nasal catarrh is first caused by inflammation of the membrane of the nasal cavities and air passages, which is followed by ulceration, when Nature, in order to protect this delicate tissue and preserve the olfactory nerves, throws a tough membrane over the ulcerated condition. At this stage it is designated chronic catarrh.

TREATMENT.

Use the "Cascade" regularly every day, with water as hot as can be borne, and guard scrupulously against taking cold. The membrane must next be removed, and for this purpose we most unhesitatingly recommend the J.B.L. Catarrh Remedy.

Half a lifetime of careful research has been devoted to perfecting this admirable preparation, which to-day stands first as an effective agent in removing this membraneous obstruction. It is composed of several kinds of oils, and gently but effectually removes the membrane that Nature has built over the inflamed parts, while its emollient character soothes and allays the inflammation. These oils are not absorbed into the system, but act only locally.

The method of application is as follows: A small quantity is placed in a glass douche (especially manufactured for the purpose) and inhaled, allowing the fluid to pass up the nostrils and into the throat, using the nostrils alternately.

There is no case of catarrh so obstinate but will readily yield to this treatment. But as a preventive of all this keep the colon clean and pay attention to lung development.

ERYSIPELAS.

This disease arises from impure blood. A peculiar poison is generated, which declares itself in the form of a red, puffy swelling, closely resembling a blister, and very much like it to the touch. If the finger is pressed upon the inflamed part, it will leave a white spot there for an instant. It most usually attacks the face and head. In the majority of cases it arises from an obstructed colon, a fermentation being generated there from the long retained faecal matter, consequently a positive and sure cure is to thoroughly cleanse that organ. As a local application take loppered sour milk and apply it to the inflamed parts, or, if not this, the next best thing is hop yeast mixed with charcoal to the thickness desired. The lactic acid in sour milk is a direct antidote to the poison of erysipelas.

DYSPEPSIA.

This disease does not come by chance. Infection or contagion can never be held responsible for it. It is the penalty which Nature inflicts upon you for violating physiological laws. Do not be deluded by extravagantly worded advertisements into the belief that any nostrum has been or ever will be invented that can possibly effect an immediate cure. You must entirely abandon the habits that induced it. You must masticate your food thoroughly--allowing the saliva to mix with it, not bolt it, and then wash it down with copious draughts of tea, coffee or water. This superabundance of fluid only serves to distend the stomach and impede digestion. A change of diet is necessary, but not so essential as a change in the habit of eating. Dyspepsia is more or less catarrh of the stomach. Its lining becomes coated with a slimy mucus that arrests the action of the glands, coats the food and prevents the gastric juice from acting upon it.

TREATMENT.

For the first week, use the "Cascade" every night, the second week, each alternate night; thereafter, as occasion seems to demand. Drink a glass of hot water, not less than half an hour before each meal, especially before breakfast. The breakfast should commence with a liberal amount of good, ripe fruit, preferably oranges or grape fruit. This may be followed by a small quantity of some good preparation of whole-wheat: possibly, a lightly boiled or poached egg and a slice of crisp, dry toast, or whole-wheat bread. Drink nothing with the food, but take a glass of hot milk half an hour later. Good, lean beef or mutton, broiled or baked, is easily digested, and may be eaten moderately at midday. If faint between meals, take a glass of hot milk, with a raw egg beaten in it. If the stomach is very sensitive, it is better to eat five or six meals a day, of a few ounces, than to overtax the stomach. Masticate every mouthful of food thoroughly, and practice deep breathing assiduously, it is an important aid to digestion. This method of treatment, if faithfully persisted in, will cure the worst case of dyspepsia, with all its attendant misery.

RHEUMATISM.

Both chronic and acute rheumatism are diseases of the blood, due to an excess of uric acid. The presence of this acid is due to excessive and imperfect action of the liver. Imperfect nutrition and deficient excretion are the primary causes, and the result is that the blood becomes loaded with poisonous matter. The trouble manifests itself in the joints, toes, ankles, knees or hands, but the seat of the disease is elsewhere.

TREATMENT.

The first thing to be done is to promote the conversion of acid by oxidation and increased activity of the liver. The best way to accomplish this is by the daily use of the "Cascade," first with hot water, then with cool water, doubling the antiseptic tonic. Do this twice a day for a week, then once a day for a month. Take a Turkish bath daily for a time to restore the functions of the skin. Rub the disabled joints with hot, oily applications, followed by massage and pressure movements. The diet should consist largely of green vegetables, mutton and whole wheat bread, or toast, eggs, milk and fruit. Avoid pastry and starchy food, such as potatoes, beans and white bread. A cup of hot water, not less than half an hour before breakfast, should not be omitted.

This treatment will speedily cure the worst cases.

TYPHOID FEVER.

The chief seat of this terribly prevalent disease is in the stomach and intestines, particularly the colon. It is a foul, bacterial disease, and originates in filth. The germs may be taken into the system in impure water or milk, inhaling the gases from defective drains or by eating food which has absorbed such gases. Once in the system, the bacteria must have decayed matter to feed upon, therefore it is impossible for a person who is clean both inside and out to take typhoid fever, there being no facilities for the germs to breed and multiply. A peculiar secretion from the colon, mixed with the faecal matter of long standing, induces a fermentation that generates a putrid smelling gas. This fermenting gas is the home of the bacillus, and from it millions of germs are multiplied and pass into the circulation. In this fermentation a peculiar worm is bred, which is the cause of ulceration in the bowels of typhoid patients.

TREATMENT.

To give physic in a typhoid fever case is a grave mistake. Instead of assisting Nature, it more probably hastens the death of the patient. Knowing the cause of the disease, common sense tells us that the first thing to do is to check the multiplication of the germs by removing the putrid matter in which they breed. When the symptoms first appear give the patient a warm water emetic. Drink until the stomach throws it back. Do not be afraid to drink. If the stomach is obstinate, use the index finger to excite vomiting. This washes out the contents of the stomach, which will be found fermenting and full of bacteria. Then give him a large cup of hot water--very hot--with a little salt in it. Let the patient rest for an hour or so after vomiting, then use the "Cascade" with water just as hot as the hand will bear, so it will not scald. Let him retain the water from ten to fifteen minutes if he can. Next, the patient must be sweated, to open up the pores of the skin, and for this nothing equals the wet sheet pack. Roll the patient in a sheet wrung out of cold water, on top of this a couple of blankets and a comfortable. At his feet place hot bricks in flannel, on his head a towel, wrung out of cold water. Give him plenty of fresh air. When he has perspired freely take him out of the pack, wash him with warm water and soap, rub him down, give him a drink of cold water and put him to bed. Repeat the injections daily, using tepid water. In cases of extreme weakness the treatment must be modified. Let the patient have all the cold water he wants to drink and give him plenty of fresh air. Use flushings daily, also the external bath, remembering in the latter to use cold water when the fever is high, and he will speedily be restored to health. Let him eat nothing until Nature calls for it. The best test of hunger is a piece of stale dry Graham bread.

BILIOUS FEVER.

This disease generally makes its appearance with one or more chills, sickness of the stomach and more or less fever. The tongue has an ill- looking yellow coat and food is unacceptable. The cause of all this, to an intelligent mind, is perfectly clear. The colon is clogged and the acids in the stomach and the duodenum, together with an abundance of secretions from the liver, have no outlet. In this condition a slight cold will close up the already overworked pores of the skin and turn the tide of corruption into the stomach, lungs and kidneys, and bilious fever is the result, for, Nature being unable to get rid of the filth by the ordinary methods, resorts to her last expedient, of burning it up.

TREATMENT.

The remedy is obviously simple. Use the "Cascade" and open the pores. Wash the stomach, take two or three hot injections daily, and a hot sheet pack. This treatment, with baths and rubbing, will cure an ordinary case of bilious fever in about three days. Avoid all drugs. Nature will call for food when it needs it.

LA GRIPPE.

This is the modern name for influenza. It resembles an ordinary cold in its symptoms, but is far more violent in its effects. Acute pains in the head and kidneys are symptoms that are usually present. If neglected, it may develop into pneumonia, or consumption. It is both epidemic and contagious, and thousands of victims were left in its trail when it swept over the United States and Europe during the winters of 1890, 1891 and 1892.

TREATMENT.

Possibly you are not aware that this disease is almost invariably accompanied by constipation, but it is a fact, nevertheless, consequently, the internal bath is the first remedial process to be resorted to. Make them hot and copious, and use them daily, for three days at least. Next, relieve the internal congestion by opening the pores of the skin. To do this, use the Turkish bath (see end of book), take it at night, drink a glass of hot lemonade, and go to bed. Tuck yourself up warm. Doubtless it will make you sweat, but you need that. In the morning take a bath and a good rub down. Drink a cup of hot water half an hour before breakfast, and let that meal consist of plain food, soft-boiled eggs, oatmeal, Graham bread and fruit-- oranges, if procurable. Two days of this treatment will put La Grippe to flight, but the better plan is to prevent it by keeping the colon cleansed.

DYSENTERY.

This is a disease of the colon. The retention of faecal matter in the folds of the colon inflames the parts until they become dry, then the soft evacuations dry on the sensitive mucous membrane. These secretions produce a peculiar acid, which in its turn breeds worms, and these, in the early stages of their existence, eat into the foreign matter and even into the mucous membrane itself, causing what is known as dysentery.

TREATMENT.

In either the acute or chronic cases, the patient must be treated lying down, with the hips elevated above the shoulders. For this purpose our Fountain attachment is necessary with the "Cascade." This will relieve the pain and congestion in the lower part of the colon. In acute cases do not let the patient sit up a moment. Use a bed pan always. Flush the colon with hot water, letting it flow gently, and add a little salt to the water. After the discharge, follow with an injection of two ounces of vaseline oil, which should be retained as long as possible. This is an emollient, and will soothe and heal the ulcerations.

During the past seven years we have been instrumental in curing uses of dysentery contracted during the Civil Ware and solely by the foregoing treatment.

DIARRHOEA

Is simply Nature's method of getting rid of undigested substances in the alimentary tract. After a time the irritation excites the glands to abnormal action to wash out the offending substances, resulting from excessive fermentation. If not relieved, ulceration sets in, and worms breed in the intestines--then we have what is known as chronic diarrhoea.

The treatment in both varieties is the same. Use the "Cascade" until the colon is thoroughly emptied and cleansed. Take a warm bath before retiring, and follow it with a brisk rub down. Be careful in your diet--the better plan being to fast for a day or two, until the worst symptoms are past.

DISEASES OF THE NERVES.

Most people imagine that nervousness is the result of too much nerve force, but the opposite is the case. The trouble is a too sensitive battery and inadequate nerve force. The batteries, or nerve centres, are too easily discharged. It is nervous irritability, therefore, that we have to deal with.

The causes are manifold, the restless American nature, the stimulating climate, neglect of physical training, giving too little time and attention to eating and sleeping, concentrating too much attention on money getting and business to the neglect of recreation and repose. One of the gravest causes is a constipated colon, which promotes indigestion, and through it, lack of nutrition, thus cutting off the supply of nerve food. The habit of tea and coffee drinking, and the use of tobacco, are also fruitful causes of this distressing affliction.

TREATMENT.

You must apply a brake to that restless motor within you that is driving you too fast. You must step out of the busy stream of life for awhile, let it rush past you and take things easy. Flush the colon regularly--remove that great source of nervous irritation, for we have yet to hear of a nervous person that was not constipated.

If you suffer from nervousness, you are dyspeptic, your whole course of life tends to render you so. Follow the treatment, especially the diet, given under the head of "Dyspepsia." Practice deep breathing, for lung development, for strong lung power is never associated with nervousness. Take plenty of exercise in the open air, but not to excess.

Be moderate in all things, except sleep, you cannot sleep too much. Cultivate the sleeping habit, and don't give up until you can sleep ten hours a day.

THE MATTER OF FOOD

is important, for, as before stated, nervous people eat and sleep too little. Fatty foods, or those that are easily converted into fat, are what is necessary. Olive oil is one of the best nerve foods in existence. Take a teaspoonful at a time, and gradually increase the quantity until you can take a tablespoonful at each meal. If you really can't take olive oil, the best substitute is sweet cream. Celery is also good, and lettuce.

Cultivate slow and measured movements, avoid undue activity, take life easy and be moderate in all things.

To sum up. Flush the colon, sleep long, eat slowly, and plenty of oily or fat food, exercise freely, but in moderation, develop the lungs by breathing exercises, and take life easy.

This line of treatment, faithfully carried out, will cure the very worst cases in time.

HEADACHE.

There are many causes for this distressing complaint. Generally the cause is to be found in the stomach. Something that has no right there is in that organ, and irritating the pneumogastric nerve that connects the stomach with the brain. It is a common symptom of dyspepsia.

An engorged colon is one of the most common causes, on the same principle that it causes paralysis and apoplexy. Stimulants invariably promote headache.

To prevent the attacks, live regularly, avoid late hours and excessive brain work, shun alcoholic beverages and tea and coffee, avoid sweets and pastries, and anything fried in fat. Eat good, plain food, including fruit (especially oranges), but never eat late at night. Develop the lungs. Never let a day pass without gently exercising all the muscles. Massage the abdomen each night before retiring. Keep the colon clean by the use of the "Cascade," and bathe at least three times a week.

To relieve an attack, flush the colon thoroughly. Take a hot foot-bath, and while taking it, take a cup of hot lemonade--without sugar--so hot that you have to sip it.

DROPSY.

In this disease the outlet to the intestinal canal has become clogged. The kidneys wear out trying to evacuate the bowels through their delicate tubular network, and the capillaries have become helpless through misuse in trying to do the work of others. So the tissues and muscles of the extremities are loaded with this cast off material, and we call it bloat. This is dropsy.

TREATMENT.

Empty and cleanse the colon with the "Cascade." Take the following injection every night, and retain it: To a pint of hot water add ten drops of the homeopathic tincture of Indian Hemp. If that is not to be had, use the fluid extract of Merrill's preparation. Use every night until a decided improvement is seen. If you do not get the desired effect, double the dose--even forty drops will do no harm. It is not a poison, but an excellent diuretic for dropsical effusions.

Take a Turkish bath (see end of book) to open up the pores of the skin, but if the patient is too weak use the hot wet sheet pack. Use the "Cascade" at least twice a week, following it with the injection mentioned above. Eat as little as possible, and let that consist of dry toast well masticated, and do not take any tea or coffee.

APPENDICITIS.

This complaint was formerly known as inflammation of the bowels, and may be caused by injury. It was generally believed to be due to the presence of foreign substances, such as grape seeds, etc., in the vermiform appendix, but this idea is exploded. It is an inflamed condition of the appendix, but the inflammation may have extended from the colon or from the peritoneum. The most frequent cause is the caecum (the lower pouch of the colon) getting filled with hardened faecal matter, in which case the ileo caecal valve is obstructed, and the natural passages of the bowels stopped. With a clean colon appendicitis is practically an impossibility.

The accepted medical practice is to remove the appendix by operation, regardless of conditions; but the mortality in such cases is high. Others put the patient to sleep with tincture of opium, or veratrum viride, and let Nature right herself, if possible. If Nature can maintain herself against the doctor and his drugs from seven to nine days, the patient may get round, but not well.

TREATMENT.

Use the "Cascade" promptly on the first sign of an attack, injecting all the water possible (at a temperature of not less than 102 Fahr.), so as to reach the caecum, where the trouble is located. If the attack is an acute one, use the "Cascade" every third hour until relieved. If the obstruction (which is usually present) does not give way, inject a pint of hot water and a pint of castor oil mixed; but before injecting it (with a bulb syringe) raise the patient's hips several inches higher than his head; then turn the patient on his right side, and stroke the reverse way of the colon, applying a firm but gentle kneading movement in the region of the appendix. This injection should be retained at least half an hour--longer if necessary. If this does not break loose the obstruction, resume the use of the "Cascade." Hot fomentations over the appendicular region are valuable. Give no medicine, it can do no good, but may do infinite mischief. After the bowel has been emptied let the patient have absolute rest, and if there is much pain and inflammation present, apply cracked ice, in a rubber bag, over the affected part. The diet should be absolutely liquid until all danger has passed. This is of the highest importance.

DISEASES OF THE LIVER.

Liver complaints are always closely related to other diseases of the digestive organs. The colon being clogged, the intestines are rendered sluggish, which in turn acts upon the duodenum, or second stomach, and prevents the food from properly passing out--then fermentation takes place. Bile is poured out on the accumulated food again and again, for the presence of anything in the duodenum is a demand for the secretion of bile. As a result too much bile is mixed with the food to be absorbed--the blood becomes tainted with biliary secretions showing itself in a yellow skin, dizziness of the head, dull, sleepy condition and lack of ambition. This overtaxing of the organ results in what is known as acute congestion, the symptoms of which are tenderness to touch and a feeling of painful tension on right side just above the edge of the ribs, slight jaundice, furred tongue, loss of appetite and scanty high colored urine.

TREATMENT.

Open the colon by the use of the "Cascade," when the intestines and duodenum will be in turn relieved, then open up the pores of the skin with baths and allow Nature to expel the waste from the system in that manner. The wet sheet pack will he found specially valuable for that purpose.

An unnatural appetite often accompanies bilious attacks, but it should be resisted. Eat sparingly of bread and milk, slightly salted, for two or three days, then take more solid food, but do not eat meat more than once a day for a week or two. Any exercises that call the muscles of the stomach into play are beneficial and should be practiced daily, especially horseback riding and rowing. Exercise by bending forward, trying to touch the toes without bending the knees; at the same time taking a deep breath--you then have the liver as in a vise, thus inducing active circulation.

The "Bear" walk, or walking about the room on all fours without bending the knees, is one of the best exercises for a torpid liver that can be imagined, but it should be practised in private, or your friends may question your sanity.

DISEASES OF THE SKIN.

These diseases usually have their origin in constipation, therefore tile first tiling to be done is to relieve this condition of the colon by daily use of the "Cascade." Bathe the body daily in tepid water, being careful not to use soap that will irritate the skin.

Never use common soap nor any of the highly perfumed varieties. A pure soap will float in the water. An occasional wet pack sheet is of great value. Attend care fully to the diet and avoid all foods fried in fat, especially buckwheat cakes and food of that description.

DISEASE OF THE KIDNEYS.

This is caused by irritation of the kidneys, brought about by those organs being forced to do work which does not properly belong to them.

Congestion is the first step towards chronic or acute inflammation. The second stage is a breaking down or degeneration of the kidney cells. If degeneration has passed a certain point, there is no hope.

TREATMENT.

The only possible cure is to remove the cause. The colon, intestines, stomach and skin must be got into good working order, so that they will do their own work and relieve the poor scapegoat the kidneys--of unjust burdens. The colon should be constantly and copiously flushed with the "Cascade," and warm baths frequently taken. The Turkish bath is valuable, especially the home bath described in this book, as the patient's head, being free, the hot air is not drawn into the lungs.

Every night after flushing the colon inject a pint of warm water and go to bed. It will pass off through the kidneys, cleansing them. If there is acute pain, repeat the injection every two hours until relieved. Hot fomentations applied to the back, over the region of the kidneys, will relieve the pain, and gentle massage in the same locality will be found beneficial.

Avoid sweets, pastries, starchy foods, like potatoes, alcohol, tobacco, tea, coffee and overfat foods. The diet recommended for dyspepsia is good. Skim milk, buttermilk and whey should be used freely, as they exercise a very beneficial influence on the kidneys. A wet compress worn over night will help draw out the poisonous waste matters.

ASIATIC CHOLERA.

This disease is caused by the presence of a microbe, known as the "comma bacillus," which manufactures a virulent poison, called a ptomaine. Although the germs are taken into the system through the medium of the mouth and stomach, they only multiply in the bowels, which is proved by the fact that the vomit from a cholera patient contains none, while the discharges from the bowels abound with them. If the system is in perfect condition the germs are destroyed by the gastric juice in the stomach as soon as inhaled. If the stomach is out of order the bacilli escape into the intestines, where the fluids are alkaline (in which they thrive) and cholera is the result. The symptoms are, first a slight diarrhcea, almost painless, then tremors, vertigo and nausea. Griping pains and repressed circulation follow, then copious purging of the intestines, followed by discharges of a thin watery fluid, lividity of the lips, cold breath and an unquenchable thirst.

TREATMENT.

First flush the colon thoroughly with warm water every few hours. Next induce perspiration by means of the Turkish bath, but if the case has set in violently, and vomiting and cramps appear, use the "Cascade" promptly, and get the patient into bed as quickly as possible. Then take two heavy sheets, dip them in water as hot as can be borne, fold them and lay them over the chest and abdomen and cover up with blankets, tucking them in closely at the sides. Put a jug of hot water to the feet. In about ten minutes redip the sheets quickly and reapply. In fifteen or twenty minutes the perspiration will appear and the cramps will vanish. Take nothing into the stomach during the duration of the disease except moderate sips of cold water or pieces of ice, to quench the burning thirst.

Use simple strengthening food (milk is best) until health is restored. All water should be boiled before using.

CHOLERA MORBUS.

The symptoms are similar to those of Asiatic cholera, but not so violent. The treatment is the same in principle. If there is a feeling of nausea take a warm water emetic.

PERITONITIS

Is an inflammation of the membrane covering the bowels, and is frequently caused by concussion or injury; sometimes it extends from adjacent organs, but in many instances it is caused by the breeding of worms in the hardened faecal accumulations in the colon.

No matter what the cause may he, flush the colon vigorously with injections as hot as can be borne, and place bags of hops, steeped in hot vinegar, on the outside. This will soon reduce the inflammation and effect a cure.

PNEUMONIA,

Sometimes called Lung Fever, is an acute inflammation of the lungs, usually caused by a cold, and commencing with a chill and feverish symptoms. At first there is a dry cough and what is known as the brick dust sputum, and in the advanced stages a peculiar dark tint in the cheeks, known as the mahogany flush. The breathing becomes very hurried, rising as high as forty respirations per minute. It is an exceedingly rapid and frequently fatal form of disease.

TREATMENT.

Promptitude in dealing with the case is of the highest importance. If the colon had been kept clean and the lungs developed by exercise it could not have attacked you; therefore the first thing to be done is to use the "Cascade." Then the circulation must be equalized by drawing the blood to the skin and extremities--away from the congested lungs. A hot foot-bath will draw the blood to the extremities and a Turkish bath (see end of book) will do the same to the skin. If too weak to endure the Turkish bath, substitute a hot bath. Put the patient to bed immediately and apply a hot compress over the lungs, wrung out of hot brine, changing it as often as it gets cool. Give little, extremities-away any, food during the continuance of the disease; if any is given it should be light and nutritious. The above treatment, if employed in time, will save any case.

BRONCHITIS.

This is an acute inflammation of the bronchial tubes, or air passages, and the treatment is almost identical with that for pneumonia; only applying the hot compress to the throat or chest, according to which part exhibits the most soreness. If the throat is very sore use the following gargle: Bichromate of potash (pulverized), one drachm; tincture capsicum, half ounce; pure water, two tablespoonfuls. Shake until dissolved. Add one teaspoonful of this mixture to three-fourths of a tumbler of water and gargle the throat every hour until relieved--then every two hours until well.

ASTHMA.

A mast distressing complaint, and hitherto imperfectly understood. It has been attributed to innumerable causes, but our contention is that it is due to an engorged transverse colon, which, interfering with the free action of the diaphragm, withdraws that amount of impetus from the lungs, so that they fail to respond to nerve stimulation. Through inaction, the diaphragm becomes practically a fixed instead of a movable partition. This contention is borne out by the fact that in numerous cases where the colon was emptied, the trouble disappeared and no trouble was experienced so long as the colon was kept clean. In all cases of asthma the last meal should be a light one, if taken at all; in fact, it would be well to follow the dietary rules for dyspepsia, and in addition omit the evening meal.

UTERINE DISPLACEMENT.

This prevalent complaint among the women of America is due, in ninety per cent. of the cases, to constipation, and that is mainly attributable to tight lacing. In the majority of our countrywomen the sigmoid flexure (see diagram beginning of work) is distended to nearly double its natural size, pressing upon the womb, which necessarily displaces it, but in addition the colon, through impaction, frequently becomes highly inflamed and communicates the inflammation to the womb, making it heavy and relaxed.

The ascending and descending colon lie immediately behind the ovaries, and if (as is often the case) it becomes distended to double its size, it stretches the broad ligaments and ovarian connections, frequently breaking them away from their peritoneal attachments or carrying the peritoneum downward with them.

The Fallopian tubes, which penetrate and are attached to the peritoneal sack, together with the uterine broad ligaments, are designed to hold the womb in place, but if the womb and ovaries are crowded down into the pelvic cavity and the womb doubled upon itself, dysmenorrhea or painful menstruation, or amenorrhea, with convulsions, is the result. Perhaps there may even be a complete stoppage, so that Nature menstruates vicariously and casts it off through the lungs or bowels.

TREATMENT.

Empty the colon and keep it clean by regular use of the "Cascade," and wear your clothing as loose as your husband's or brother's, and the womb will go back into its place, and all the bad symptoms disappear. It may be, though, that the tendons and ligaments have become partially paralyzed through the uterus having been so long out of place.

After emptying the colon, if there is pain in the back, with a bearing down sensation, sit in half a tub of hot water for fifteen or twenty minutes once every other day. Throw yourself on your back with the hips raised as high as possible, then rub up from the pelvic bone. This will reduce the displacement of the sigmoid flexure, besides giving relief. Should the womb not go back into place, call in a physician to replace it.

Painful menstruation and leucorrhea, which are caused by displacement of the womb, inflammation and hypertrophy, or hardening of the womb, enlarged and sensitive ovaries, can all be speedily cured by flushing the colon.

ANTEVERSION,

Which affects nine out of every ten women, is the womb falling forward on the bladder (causing frequent desire to urinate) and downward, which, with the falling of the sigmoid flexure, produces obstruction of the bowels and great straining at stool.

RETROVERSION

Is a falling down, with the body of the womb thrown backward. Frequently it is doubled upon itself, when it becomes hardened and inflamed, and adhesion often takes place. Doctors frequently call this spinal disease, but it is the displaced organs pressing on the great sympathetic nerve, which produces partial paralysis of the lower limbs and loss of memory, sometimes causing insanity. In retroversion, after emptying the colon, assume the following position: Kneel on the bed, or sofa, with the body thrown forward until the chest also touches. Retain this position as long as possible, and repeat it frequently during the day. Sleep with the foot of the bed raised eight inches. These positions all facilitate the return of the womb to its normal position.

Eat nutritious, easily digested food, and avoid all stimulants.

COMMON COLDS

Are very disagreeable things, and, though not dangerous in themselves, yet are frequently the cause of serious complications and the forerunners of consumption, pneumonia and catarrh. Colds are commonly due to sudden changes of temperature, and are caused by the sudden closing of the pores of the skin, thus preventing the escape of those waste matters of the body which Nature has designed should be expelled in that direction. The blood is thus driven inward, causing congestion. If the system is in a sound, healthy condition, with respiration good and the colon clean, it should be next to impossible to take cold. If, however, there is a weak spot in the body, be sure the cold will find it, when, if not promptly dealt with, serious results may ensue.

TREATMENT.

Constipation is the invariable primary cause of a cold, hence the first thing to do is to flush the colon. Use the "Cascade" daily for at least three days. Do not eat any supper the first night. The next thing to be done is to take the Turkish bath (see end of book). It should be taken at night, after which drink a glass of hot lemonade and go to bed, covering the body thoroughly. No doubt you will perspire profusely, but that is what you need. In the morning take a good bath and rub down, following the directions given for bathing, drink a cup of hot water an hour before breakfast and let that meal be light, such as Graham bread, boiled eggs, oatmeal and oranges. You are then ready to attend to your daily business, and if you take another flushing at night, the next morning your cold will be only a memory.

CONSTIPATION.

This condition of the system has been so frequently referred to already that further comment upon it may be deemed unnecessary. Its causes are varied, insufficient exercise in the open air, hastily eaten and imperfectly masticated food, also many articles of food tend to induce the evil of habitual constipation.

Whatever you may do, avoid everything in the form of drugs, for they are injurious in the highest degree. The continual excitation of the excretory processes by the use of cathartics is a most pernicious practice and should be shunned. A constant indulgence in the "purgative habit" often renders the coating of the stomach so sensitive that even the presence of food in that organ irritates it and is frequently hurried out half digested.

The "Cascade" should be used each alternate day, for at least two weeks, then, twice a week, until improvement is assured. Drink a tumblerful of hot water, not less than half an hour before breakfast and eat freely of fruit at that meal. Also partake liberally of good, green vegetables at other meals. Eating whole-wheat bread is of decided assistance, and make it a rule to drink from two to three pints of water each day.

PILES OR HEMORRHOIDS.

This is a disease of the rectum and muscles of the anus, and is the direct result of constipation. The accumulation of hardened faecal matter distends the sigmoid flexure, causing inflammation, until from its own weight it falls down, producing prolapse of the bowels. Frequently ulceration follows and the bowel is pressed out, tumors forming on the protruding portion.

Bleeding piles are caused by congestion of the rectal blood vessels. The constant nerve irritation causes muscular contraction, consequently circulation is interfered with, producing a condition of engorgement. Owing to lack of nutrition the structures become brittle and quantities of the varicosed capillaries unite to form pile tumors. The methods of treatment usually employed are, injecting astringents into the tumors to dry them up; to ligate the tumors, that they may die or drop off, or to amputate the portion of the rectum in which the tumors form (known as the radical operation), none of which prevent a return of the trouble. The only rational plan is to remove the cause.

TREATMENT.

First empty the colon, using the "Cascade," thus removing the cause, then the inflammation will subside and the protruding bowel go back into its place. Tumors will soon absorb if they are put back when they protrude. Sitting in a tub of hot water will cause the bowel to go back immediately. Hot water is Nature's astringent and never fails. The following salve has been found of great value in facilitating recovery: Two heaped tablespoonfuls of vaseline or cosmoline, willow charcoal, one teaspoonful; canadies pinus canadensis, twenty-five drops; sulphate morphia, five grains. Mix well and apply up the rectum with the fingers as far as possible. But the most effective aid to a cure is to follow the use of the "Cascade," by inserting in the rectum a small piece of ice, about the size of the tip of the little finger (previously immersed in water to render it smooth), which will be found a most admirable rectal tonic, driving the blood away from the congested parts, and producing a bracing effect on the structures. In bad cases, it may be used with good effect several times during the day, and will be found equally beneficial in cases of prolapse of the rectum. The ice is to be retained in the rectum.

PARALYSIS OR PALSY.

These two terms signify one and the same disease; that is, a condition of the system in which the power of voluntary motion is lost. It is the outward manifestation of a deep-seated disease that can usually be traced to an obstructed colon and consequent disordered circulation. The same causes promote apoplexy. A blood vessel is ruptured in the brain, causing a clot to form, which presses upon the nerves that convey the will of the mind to the muscles, thus stopping their action. It is not, as is usually supposed, an affection of the muscles, but of the nerves that control the muscular movements. Sometimes one entire side of the body becomes affected and completely deprived of voluntary motion. Congestion of the brain is a preliminary of paralysis, and congestion of the brain are invariably due to an enlarged transverse colon.

One form of paralysis affects only certain parts of the body, such. as the lower limbs, or the reproductive organs, and is caused by pressure upon some large nerve communicating with the paralyzed portion. This is doubtless due to the pressure of an enlarged ascending or descending colon upon some of the lumbar plexus nerves, or their branches. This, however, refers to what may be termed local paralysis, or paralysis of certain parts.

Paralysis of an entire side of the body is due to pressure on the brain, and this is caused by defective circulation, induced by an unnaturally distended colon. While in this condition some severe physical exertion or mental strain increases the pressure beyond the power of resistance and a rupture is the result--when the patient falls, wherever he may happen to be.

TREATMENT.

Prevention of paralysis is very easy, for with a clean colon it is an impossibility, and the remedy is too plainly indicated to need pointing out. You have but to remove the cause--the accumulation in the colon. Massage is a most valuable part of the treatment. To prevent the muscles from stiffening, and to retain the suppleness of the affected parts, frequent rubbings are necessary, and the mind should be stimulated to resume its control over the refractory muscles. During an attack it is necessary to pay particular attention to diet-- easily digested, nonconstipating food only. You may have to revert to a spoon diet for awhile--and, as the liability to a second attack is great during the period of recovery, special attention must be given to diet to guard against it.

When power begins to return to the affected parts, a system of graduated exercises should be arranged, gradually increasing in force with the return of strength and normal control. These exercises will gradually educate the mind and restore its harmonious working with the body.

EPILEPSY, OR FALLING SICKNESS,

Is distinguished from apoplexy, or paralysis, by the convulsive action and foaming at the mouth. One prime cause of this most distressing complaint is the action of worms in the colon. In a number of cases treated by us, knots of worms were expelled, and the exciting cause being removed, complete recovery followed. The preventive treatment is simple. Use the "Cascade" and out antiseptic tonic until the worms are entirely expelled. During a fit loosen the clothing at the throat and place something in the mouth, a cork, for instance, to prevent the patient from biting his tongue. Some fine salt thrust into the mouth will shorten the duration of the fit.

Another prolific cause is masturbation, in which case nothing but the abandonment of the habit and a cleanly life, both physically and morally, will effect a cure.

GONORRHEA.

This is a contagious disease, and its victims usually become the prey of unprincipled charlatans, who drive the disease inward by suppressing the symptoms. It affects the male much more seriously than the female. It commences with a slight uneasy sensation at the mouth of the urethra, between the second and seventh day after exposure to infection. The natural discharge of mucus is increased, and is more viscid, followed by acute inflammation. The discharge becomes thick and greenish and urination is painful. Swelling of the glands in the groin is common, called a bubo. Orchitis or swelling of the testicle is also a frequent accompaniment. Under the best of treatment it will require from four to six weeks to effect a cure, but if neglected it may mean months.

TREATMENT.

Use the "Cascade" every night for the first two weeks, then twice a week for at least two months, to get the poison out of the system, and keep the parts scrupulously clean by bathing them two or three times a day. Carefully avoid everything in the form of a stimulant, especially alcoholic drinks, also tobacco, and let the diet be largely vegetable. Use the following injection twice every day after urinating. Colored fluid hydrastis, two drachms; fluid extract canadies pinus canadensis, two drachms; bromo chiorellum, half a drachm; water, six ounces. Shake well and inject twice a day until a marked improvement can be noticed, then once a day, and, finally, every other day.

HERNIA OR RUPTURE

Is the escape of some portion of the viscera through an abnormal opening and takes its particular name from the locality in which the protrusion occurs, although the inguinal is the most common form. The dynamic force of foul gases engendered in the system is a prolific, though generally unsuspected cause; but the mechanical pressure exerted by an overloaded colon in the limited space of the abdominal cavity is responsible for seventy-five per cent, of all cases. The treatment is obvious--use the "Cascade" faithfully, and, the cause being removed, reduction is easy, and if the colon be kept clean, a properly adjusted truss will soon completely cure it.

INEBRIETY

Is responsible for many of the ills of the present generation, in the form of transmitted constitutional weakness, not to mention the functional derangements and organic destruction, of which it is a potent and direct cause.

There are two grave reasons why alcohol should not be taken into the system, or, if at all, in very minute quantities and at distant intervals. The first is the moral reason, because it undermines and destroys the finer part of man. It has the peculiar effect upon the brain of stimulating the baser qualities and blunting the finer ones. The second is the physical reason, see "The Diet Question." When alcoholism becomes a fixed habit, it must be treated as a disease, for it is one in reality. In many cases the large intestinal or tapeworm is at the root of the trouble. Now, worms cannot exist in a perfectly clean body, with every function working properly. Few, if any, animals can resist the solvent power of the gastric juice if it is secreted in normal quantity, and in full health and vigor, consequently, to cleanse the body of all superabundant filth and restore it to a sound working condition, will prevent their growth. But if they are present and developed (as they sometimes are) to an enormous size, the vital forces are unable to dislodge them, unaided, and recourse must be bad to a "vermifuge" diet. This may be found in two articles--the crusts of good, sweet wheat-meal bread and good, ripe uncooked apples. It is important that the food be hard, so that it be well masticated and that it be eaten slowly, so that the stomach is not overloaded.

TREATMENT.

First get the alcohol out of the system by flushing the colon daily. This will help you to stop drinking (which is so much easier advised than accomplished), then proceed to sweat it out by a daily Turkish bath (see end of book) or a Turkish bath one day and a wet sheet pack the next.

Second, sip a cupful of hot water not less than half an hour before each meal and use the wheat bread crusts and apple diet mentioned before for one week certain, two weeks is better (if possible). Then use the "cascade" thoroughly, to expel the worm; and for a month at least follow the diet laid down for dyspepsia, when the alcoholized blood in your veins will have been replaced with good, rich blood, and your cure practically effected.

OBESITY.

The condition of the body, to which nosologists have applied this term, is that of general engorgement, or, over-fullness, and is the result of excessive eating, or imperfect deputation, or both. Over-eating and inactivity are the chief producing causes. It is the especial prerogative of children to be fat, but when too great an accumulation comes, with advancing years, it brings discomforts, disadvantages, and oftentimes fatal diseases, among which are Apoplexy, Fatty Liver, Diabetes, Bright's Disease and Fatty Heart. The sanguine or entonic variety is distinguished by florid skin, full strong pulse, turgid veins, with firm and vigorous muscular fibres, and the serous or atonic, is denoted by a full, but frequent and feeble pulse, smooth and soft skin, plump but inexpressive figure, and general languor or debility of the vital functions.

TREATMENT.

Use the "Cascade" regularly, and take as much exercise as is possible without fatigue. A brisk three mile walk daily will work wonders in reducing weight, especially if you perspire freely. Drink a pint of hot water an hour before each meal and half an hour before retiring, to wash the sour ferments and bile from the stomach before eating and sleeping. Live principally on roast or broiled meat, fish, poultry or game, boiled rice, green vegetables, and brown bread. When people are unable to take the necessary amount of exercise, the dieting process, known as the "Salisbury system," is very effective. This consists of the lean part of good beef, from which every particle of fat and sinew is removed, then chopped to a pulp, made into small cakes and broiled-- then eaten hot. The reduction of adipose tissue demands a certain amount of self-sacrifice, but the above method, if faithfully followed, never fails to effect the purpose.

LOST MANHOOD

Is the term now generally employed to describe impotence, or physical inability to perform the sexual function. It is frequently due to conjugal excesses, but the principal cause is the baneful widespread practice of masturbation, or self-pollution. It manifests itself in what is known as Spermatorrhea, or involuntary emissions of the seminal fluid, and if allowed to continue unchecked, speedily depletes the vitality of the sufferer, and renders him a physical wreck. Do not be deceived by the lying advertisements of unprincipled charlatans, that any drug can help you. The treatment must be hygienic and thorough, and may necessitate a change in your whole mode of life.

TREATMENT.

Firstly, the colon must be kept clean, as the faecal accumulations there irritate the sensitive nerves. So it is advisable to use the "Cascade" every night for two weeks at least, then every second night. Secondly, practice the breathing and bodily movements described under the head of Exercise, and take all the exercise you can in the open air, as these things are important factors in strengthening the nervous system and hastening a cure. Thirdly, special attention must be paid to diet. If you can practice strict vegetarianism for a time, so much the better, choosing those articles most easily digested. Only plain roast or boiled beef should be eaten (if any meat be taken at all), shun all hot condiments, also tea, coffee, tobacco and alcohol-- especially the latter, for nothing can help you while you use these articles. Fourthly, after flushing, take a cold bath every night, or, if this is impracticable, bathe the genital organs, and the spine (up to the base of the brain) in cold water, and rub down vigorously with a crash towel. Fifthly, resolutely form cleanly habits of mind, as well as body; take up a course of good reading to occupy the mind, and divert it into healthy channels, and shun all reading of a sensational nature. Sixthly, avoid thinking impure and lascivious thoughts, and do not allow your mind to dwell upon your condition, but cultivate self- control. The above treatment has cured hundreds of bad cases, and will cure you, if steadily persevered in, but a strict abstinence from sexual indulgence, and an absolute abandonment of the pernicious vice, is an indispensable condition.

Frequently quite aged men write us, complaining of their sexual disability-- to all such, we say that the restoration of lost power after fifty years of age is in the highest degree improbable, and after the grand climacteric (63) is passed--it is practically impossible.

DIABETES OR DIABETES MELLITUS

Is a peculiar and troublesome disease, characterized by an excessive discharge of urine, which is heavily charged with grape sugar, which is the saccharine principle of grapes and honey, hence the term mellitus. This substance is manufactured in excess by the body, and eliminated by the kidneys. The discharge of urine is abnormally large, sometimes reaching as high as several gallons daily. Owing to the presence of sugar in the blood and the secretions, nutrition is affected, and other disturbances manifest themselves in the system. It is a disease, which, if not taken in time, usually proves fatal, and it therefore behooves the individual to keep the body in thorough order, and to carefully watch any abnormality in the urine.

TREATMENT.

The "Cascade" should be used regularly, also the wet sheet pack, to promote the action of the skin, for that organ usually exhibits a marked dryness; and its temperature should be varied to suit that of the body. If fairly vigorous, the morning cold bath should be used, for its tonic qualities, or, if weak, then the tepid bath, followed, in either case, by a brisk rubbing, to promote circulation. Diet is most important. All sweets and starchy foods, which are converted into sugar by digestion, should be shunned, while whole wheat bread, lean beef, mutton and fish, together with salads made from herbs, should be eaten. Acid fruits, such as oranges and lemons, are beneficial. Soft boiled eggs and milk (in moderation) may be taken. All food should be eaten slowly and a little at a time. The only drink should be pure water, and that never at meal times, but a cup of hot water half an hour before meals will be found of service. Tea, coffee, cream, and especially alcoholic drinks, must be absolutely avoided.

LOCOMOTOR ATAXIA

Results from what is known as sclerosis, a hardening of the gray matter in the motor centres of the spinal cord. Its special symptom is the peculiar high-stepping gait, the power of locomotion not being properly under the control of the will, and when the eyes are closed, it seems impossible for the afflicted person to walk forward without falling. Like other diseases of its class, it is primarily due to innutrition, the result of imperfect elimination, and has hitherto defied regular medical treatment. If a cure is to be effected, it is by regular use of the "Cascade," perfect rest, strict attention to diet, and judicious massage; but if the case is well advanced, it is doubtful whether restoration to health can be affected.

NURSING MOTHERS.

Under the above heading, we class the following troublesome complaints: Inflammation of the Breast, Milk Fever, Sore Nipples, Puerperal Swelled Leg, and Puerperal Fever, or Peritonitis, all of which complaints are practically unknown, under intelligent hygienic treatment.

We would point out that a simple hygienic mode of life (including careful diet and the regular practice of the "Cascade Treatment" during pregnancy), will not only have the effect of making the labor easy, and the recovery rapid, but will almost preclude the possibility of any of the above complaints manifesting themselves.

During pregnancy the "Cascade Treatment" should be regularly used twice a week, by which means the absorption of the poisonous waste matters of the system into the circulation is completely avoided, and the future health of the infant assured. The body should be bathed daily, or, if impracticable, then a brisk rubbing from head to foot, with a towel, and exercise--more or less--taken every day. The diet should consist largely of vegetables and fruit, especially after the fourth month, avoiding farinaceous foods as much as possible, such as wheat, peas, beans, barley, and especially fine wheaten flour. These foods contain the bony constitutents, and their avoidance tends to deossify the systems of both mother and child, and make childbirth what Nature intended it to be, a comparatively painless proceeding.

Careful attention to the foregoing hygienic mode of life, during pregnancy, will effectually prevent the appearance of those distressing complaints (before mentioned), pecu1iar to Nursing Mothers.

INFLAMMATION OF THE BREAST

Would never occur, if the "Cascade" had been regularly used, and the treatment for it, when present, is to use the "Cascade" thoroughly, and apply cool wet clothes, well covered with dry ones, to the breasts. If there is a surplus of milk, draw it off with the breast pump, or the more convenient method--the mouth.

SORE NIPPLES

Do not require anything but a little cream or olive oil applied to them, with occasional applications of cold, wet cloths when they are hot and painful, and occasional fomentations when they are cracked and sore--but do not fail to "flush the colon."

MILK FEVER

Is principally due to over-heated, or ill-ventilated rooms, and should be treated by at once flushing the colon, and if the patient is not too weak, use the wet sheet pack, otherwise tepid ablutions should be frequently used.

PUERPERAL SWELLED LEG

Should be treated as an acute inflammation. The colon should be thoroughly flushed, the wet sheet pack or tepid bath used frequently, and cold wet compresses applied to the afflicted limb. The patient may drink cold water freely, and the diet should consist mainly of Indian or wheat-meal gruel.

FISTULA.

There are two distinctly recognized forms of fistula, the complete and the incomplete: the latter, having only one opening, either external or internal; if the opening is internal, it is termed, "blind fistula." The complete fistula has two openings, usually, one external and one internal, but in some cases, both openings are external. Fistula is almost invariably the sequel to a neglected abscess, therefore, any form of gathering in the buttocks, should be promptly attended to. Fistula may result from an injury; but the large majority of cases are due to a congested or diseased condition of the sigmoid flexure and rectum.

TREATMENT.

It need scarcely be said, that scrupulous care and cleanliness are indispensable factors in promoting recovery, therefore, the colon must be kept absolutely clean, by the use of the "Cascade" and the parts `thoroughly bathed with warm water, at least, once daily, and the pipe of the fistula should be thoroughly cleaned three times a day, with the following solution: To half a cupful of warm water, add twenty- five drops of fluid hydrastis and one teaspoonful of finely pulverized willow charcoal. This should be mixed thoroughly and injected into the opening of the fistula, the whole of it, with a small piston syringe. If the opening is not external, then, double the quantity should be injected into the rectum. This practice should be persisted in until the discharge ceases. In some cases, operations are absolutely necessary. All stimulants should be avoided and all highly seasoned foods.

DISEASES OF CHILDREN.

The following simple methods of treating the ailments of childhood will be found remarkably efficacious, easy of application, and may be used with confidence.

CROUP.

This disease often runs in families, and is most frequently caused by sudden alterations of temperature. The symptoms are usually a harsh cough, hoarseness, sore throat, and slight fever. A croupy child needs watching. To prevent it, keep the colon clean.

The treatment cannot be too prompt. Use the "Cascade" quickly, and place the child immediately in a hot bath, and rub the lower limbs thoroughly. Wring a cloth out of cold water, and place it on the throat and chest, covering it with a thick flannel to exclude the air. Change the cloth as often as it gets dry.

SCARLET FEVER.

This is a bacillus disease. The colon being clogged, Nature is trying to cast out the impurities by way of the pores of the skin, and when these become congested we have fever. First flush the colon, then use the hot sheet pack (see end of book), if the fever is not very high, or if the child has chills. If the fever is high, use the cold sheet pack. With this treatment the rash will soon come out, and the child be easy. If fever appears again, give another injection and a sponge bath. Feed the body with water outside, and give it all it wants to drink. Give no food until Nature calls for it, then a raw egg beaten in milk. When the appetite comes back, give soft-boiled rice, or oatmeal with milk. Keep a cool head, and this treatment will save your child.

CHOLERA INFANTUM

Is a disease that can be readily cured by flushing the colon--adding a little antiseptic tonic to the water. It is purely a disease of the alimentary canal, consequently, cleansing that passage affords relief. A tepid bath, covering the legs and abdomen, is of wonderful benefit when fever is present. Be very particular with the diet. A raw egg, well beaten, in boiled milk is very nourishing.

DIPHTHERIA

Is a terribly fatal complaint, the result of a poison or germ produced in the body during the illness. The symptoms being difficult to identify, all cases of sore throat, if accompanied by fever, loss of strength, and white spots on the tonsils, should be regarded as diphtheretic.

Give full hot water flushings twice or four times every twenty-four hours. If the throat is of a grayish color, add a teaspoonful of borax to every quart of water. If it is of a dark red color, add a teaspoonful of acetic acid to every quart of water. If the child cannot retain it, place it in a hot hip bath, and then it will. After the discharge, induce perspiration with the hot sheet pack (if chilly), if not, in the cold pack, and apply a cold compress to the throat. Give the child all the cold, pure water it wants.

To treat the throat locally, take equal parts of fine salt, borax and common soda, pulverize, mix well, and by means of a quill blow well down the throat, using one quarter or half a teaspoonful.

SMALL-POX.

Is a very contagious eruptive fever, caused by a bacillus and fever, with aching of the limbs, in from nine to twelve germ peculiar to the disease. It commences with chills days after exposure.

After forty-eight hours the eruption usually appears. When rightly treated, it is not a dangerous disease.

In the case of a young person or child, the treatment is the same as for scarlet fever. Let the patient have all the water it wants in frequent drinks--a little cold water at a time.

After the eruption appears, no further treatment is necessary, except a daily flushing of the colon and a daily sponge bath in tepid water. If there is pain in the head, apply a cold compress. There is no appetite during the progress of the disease, but when the stomach demands food, great care should be exercised. Milk may be given safely. When strength returns, toasted Graham bread, mush, boiled or broiled chicken may be given.

TO PREVENT POCKMARKS.

The marking is caused by exposure to dry air and light, therefore paint the hands and face with a mixture of glycerine and charcoal--the glycerine keeps the skin soft, and the charcoal shuts out the light. It should be washed off every morning, and re-applied. Under no circumstances must the patient be allowed to scratch off the pocks.

MEASLES

Is an eruptive disease peculiar to children, slightly contagious, but not dangerous. It may commence with a slight chill, or not. The fever is usually attended with a slight cold, swollen watery eyes, and sneezing.

The first thing to be done is to bring out the rash, which is quickly done, by flushing the colon, followed by a wet sheet pack, as in scarlet fever. When the eruption is out, nothing is needed but to keep the colon clean, and wash down daily with tepid water. In all eruptive diseases guard against taking cold--for a cold closes the pores of the skin, shutting up Nature's vent through which she is expelling the disease germs.

WORMS IN THE INTESTINES.

This exceedingly prevalent and troublesome complaint may be quickly and effectually relieved by colon injections, coupled with the J. B. L. antiseptic tonic. It should be retained until the preparation has time to destroy or loosen the hold of the worms. Its action may be greatly accelerated by rubbing and churning the bowels.

INFANTILE CONVULSIONS OR FITS.

These spasms sometimes indicate the approach of one of the eruptive fevers, but usually the cause is the irritation of teething, or worms in the intestines. Although the appearance of a child under such conditions is painful, yet the danger is much less than appears.

Get the little sufferer into a hot bath as quickly as possible, and draw the blood to the skin, which will afford relief. Next, direct your attention to the bowels. If, as is exceedingly likely, worms are the cause, treat as for worms.

GALL STONES

Are the result of arrested secretion of bile, usually through congestion of the liver. Then the substances that form bile accumulate and solidify in granules. Hundreds of these continually pass off through the bowels unnoticed; but prolonged congestion causes them to cohere and form larger masses, that, in passing through the bile duct, cause intense pain, which is sometimes mistaken for appendicitis.

TREATMENT.

It is only in passing, that their presence becomes known, when all that can be done is, to favor their passage by copious fomentations of hot water and diligent use of the "Cascade." Sometimes it is impossible for the stone to pass, when it has to be removed surgically. The regular use of the "Cascade" will prevent their formation. At the first symptoms of pain in the region of the liver, follow the directions for treatment of that organ, especially the exercises, and drink freely of olive oil.

MASSAGE, SHEET-PACKS, ETC.

MASSAGE,

Which is the application of motion and pressure to the body, is a most important factor in preserving or restoring health. It affords a sick person all the benefit to be obtained from exercise without the physical effort, which he is unable to exert. The sweat glands, capillaries, and lymph channels, which constitute thousands of miles of tubing, in the body of a grown person, are, by carefully and systematically applied massage, stimulated to action. The currents in these vessels are a necessity of life. When they are obstructed, weakness is the result; when they cease, decay and death ensue.

When we rub our hands or feet, we say the friction warms them; in reality it is the inner vessels which are stimulated, and bring more warm blood to the parts. If this process is extended over the whole available surface of the body, the most beneficial results will follow.

There are three recognized methods of application. First--Rubbing, to stimulate the skin to action. Second--Rolling, and pinching gently, also a kneading movement, used principally to stimulate. the stomach, bowels, and muscular tissues. Third--Percussion, or tapping with the ends of the fingers, softly-most effiacious in stimulating the action of the lungs.

Rub the surface first with a little palm oil, or vaseline. Use the tapping movement for the chest and back, the rubbing movement for the stomach and bowels, and the pinching or kneading movement for the limbs. In dyspepsia and constipation, great benefit is derived from massage treatment of the stomach and colon--starting the movements in the right groin, where the colon commences, and following its course to its rectal extremity, (consult diagram). For rheumatism, sprains, etc., commence with hot oily applications.

Most people find massage treatment to have a gentle, soothing effect. Nearly all find their appetite increased.

THE STOMACH BATH.

The first method is simplicity itself, and consists in drinking from half to a pint of hot water, as hot as can be drank with comfort, in the morning after rising, or half an hour before breakfast. It loosens up the mucus in the stomach, and in half an hour it will have passed out.

The second consists in drinking tepid water until nauseated, then the stomach will throw it back, with its contents. This thoroughly empties and cleanses the stomach. From a pint to a quart is usually sufficient, although two quarts will do no harm. If the stomach does not reject it readily, thrust the forefinger down the throat to the end of the glottis.

The third method is by the stomach tube.

THE TURKISH BATH.

Provide a wooden bottomed Chair, and having stripped the patient of all Clothing, except a pair of woolen drawers to protect his legs from the heat, let him sit on it, with his feet ankle deep in a hot foot bath, just as hot as he can bear. Wrap him about first with a blanket, tucking it close around the neck, but letting it hang loose over the chair and vessel containing the foot bath, but so arranged as to exclude the air from his person. Over the blanket wrap one or two heavy comfortables, the object being to prevent the escape of the heat and exclude the outside air from the body. Raising one side of the comfortables and blanket, place under the chair an old tea cup half full of alcohol. Set it on fire and again close the opening. Give him a drink of cold water, and if the head feels oppressed, apply a wet towel wrung from cold water. Add more hot water to the foot bath once or twice, keeping it as hot as he can bear it during the continuance of the bath. Keep him in the bath until the alcohol is all burned out. Then wash him down with soap and tepid water, sponge off with cool water, rubbing the flesh and working the muscles vigorously the meanwhile. Then dry off by patting the skin with the towel (not rubbing it), leaving a little moisture on it; dress quickly and let him lie down for an hour or put him to bed.

It should not be taken either immediately before or after a meal. There are excellent bath cabinets to be obtained, but in their absence the above will be found excellent.

THE WET SHEET-PACK.

Spread over the bed or cot two or more heavy cornfortables, over these a pair of blankets, then, if for a person of strong vitality, wring a sheet out of cold water just dry enough not to drip, and spread it over the blanket; lay the patient stripped of all clothing on the sheet with his arms by his sides, tuck the sheet around him, then the blankets and comfortables, leaving his head out but tucking it close around the neck and over his feet--making a mummy of him, so to say. If the head is hot or aches, apply a towel wrung from cold water and renew it as often as it gets warm. To the feet apply a jug of hot water. Let him lie in the pack from twenty to forty minutes, or even longer if he is comfortable. He will soon get warm and sweat freely. This is the end desired. If he goes to sleep, as is often the case, don't be in a hurry to wake him up. He will take no harm so long as he keeps warm. See that there is plenty of fresh air in the room. When he has been in the pack a sufficient length of time close the windows, then take him out and wash him down thoroughly with soap and soft, tepid water, then sponge off with cooler water, rubbing him down vigorously and working the flesh the meanwhile. If not too weak he should assist in this operation. Then dry off by patting the skin with the towel (not rubbing it), leaving a little moisture on the skin. Then, if in the day time, and the weather is not too cold, a little exercise in the open air will be beneficial. If he is too weak to exercise put him to bed again.

Before and during the pack let him have all the cold water he wants to drink, in small quantities at a time. If the patient has but little vitality, wring the sheet out of tepid water instead of cold water.

The hot sheet-pack is used in the same manner, the only difference being that the sheet is wrung out of water as hot as can be borne.

CARE OF THE "CASCADE."

What is worth having is worth taking care of; and the "Cascade" is so likely to be called into emergency service, that it should be always in order--hence the following suggestions:

After using it, hang it up by the eyelet, until it ceases to drip; then put in the stopper. The small amount of moisture left in will help to keep it flexible. It should be kept hanging, if possible, as folds in the rubber predispose it to crack. It should be kept in an even temperature, neither too hot nor too cold.

Never pour boiling, or very hot water into it--it is not designed to withstand such a degree of heat, and do not let grease, in any form, come in contact with it, as grease decomposes rubber.

PART NINE.

SOME HELPFUL SUGGESTIONS.

If there is one thing in particular that I desire to impress upon my readers, it is, don't dread disease. It is a beneficial agent, for it is Nature's method of re-adjusting matters in the human economy. There are only two conditions, health and disease. Mark the etymology of the word! Whenever there is any departure from the normal, it is bound to manifest itself in the organ or structure most in need of repair; but as disease is a tearing down, and its cure a process of building up, it does not need the wisdom of Solomon to recognize the fact that all assistance toward recovery must come from within. Disease is just as natural a condition as health; both are the result of the operation of natural law. Disease, being Nature's method of cure, any attempt to suppress it must of necessity invite disaster.

This is one of the chief reasons why I am opposed to drug medication, because its sole aim seems to be the suppression of symptoms. Pain, the chief symptom, is not disease, but simply the messenger bringing warning of the disease to the brain. To silence this messenger, yet leave the disease unchecked, is folly. It would be just as reasonable, if the house were on fire, to cut the cord of the alarm bell, and to conclude because you could no longer hear the bell that the danger was past. Disease, therefore, being beneficial, should be welcomed as a friend, and every assistance given to Nature to assist her in restoring normal conditions.

Prevention is better than cure, you will all agree, and the great elements of prevention are, knowledge of self, cleanliness, physical, mental and moral; hygiene and sanitation. I contend that physiology is the most important subject that can engage the attention of the individual. Nothing is so essential as a knowledge of the functioning of the body in which he dwells, for it is the vehicle through which the real self is to find expression; through which he is to achieve success or failure, according to the condition of its mechanism.

No engineer can obtain from the machine under his control the highest results, unless every part of the mechanism is in perfect working order. How much more important, then, that the human organism should be in perfect adjustment, since through it the mentality is to find its highest expression? Without a knowledge of its construction and its working principles, how is the individual to raise the human machine to the highest plane of excellence and maintain it there? No one is allowed to run an engine without first passing an examination, which necessitates a certain amount of study and knowledge of the laws of mechanics; yet men undertake to run that complex machine, the human body, in utter ignorance of physiological law! Is it any wonder that there are so many breakdowns? What I contend for is the study of the fundamental facts concerning the ordinary functions of the body: of diet, dress and exercise in their relation to health, and the relative effects of good and bad air upon the system. It is of infinitely more consequence to understand the basic principles of digestion and the proper combination of foods, or to understand thoroughly the baneful effects of sleeping in a badly ventilated room, than to be the greatest living expert in conic sections. Practical physiology is the crying need of the times, especially for our children, if we expect them to be well developed--mentally morally and physically.

With such an equipment of knowledge the individual is prepared to withstand the wear and tear of life, and I may remark here that it is the tear more than the wear that figures in physical breakdown. All human beings are not endowed alike with nervous force; it is largely a matter of heredity, but what we have may be cultivated and developed. Failure to do so renders the individual liable to nervous breakdown, or neurasthenia, as it is popularly termed, a widespread disease, especially in America, where the strain of life is greater than elsewhere. Competition, a desire to go beyond one's fellows in achievement, working beyond the strength, together with lack of care of the physical system, all conspire to keep constant the undue excitement of the nerves that ends in exhaustion. Children born of nervous parents, with weak nervous systems, should be fortified against the risks of inheritance by hygienic measures, during their developmental period, strengthening in every way their physical and mental endowments. Even those well developed in this respect should husband his or her resources--always keeping a reserve fund by avoiding undue fatigue, spending plenty of time in sleep, taking care of the body, and arranging for intervals of rest that shall include change of scene and environment.

Remember that mind and thought have their effect on the bodily health, no less than material and physical conditions; and that although a healthy body needs a sane mind, it is none the less true that a sane mind needs a healthy body; therefore maintain perfect equilibrium between the two. It may surprise you to hear your body compared to a bank; but the analogy is perfect, as I shall proceed to show. No living organism is precisely the same for sixty consecutive minutes. There are perpetually losses from within and gains from without; losses in the form of broken down tissue, gains in the form of food or air, which is the most essential form of food. So, in a bank, there is a constant interchange of deposits and withdrawals. No bank could exist if the depositors insisted upon their money being hoarded up there. It is the money, and not the bank, that is the fixed consideration, money being the medium of exchange. In the human system, food is the medium, and for the same reason that a bank cannot exist by hoarding up money, it is impossible for a living organism to exist by simply storing up food. There must be a continual interchange, otherwise the human bank cannot pay dividends in the form of health and energy.

And even as some banks, that appear solid and substantial from the outside, may be on the verge of ruin, owing to the lack of supervision over income and expenditure; so many apparently robust bodies may be on the verge of physical collapse, owing to the mistaken belief that the body is simply a depository for food. Energy may be stored up in the system for future use, that being the dividend resulting from judicious interchange; but to force the system to receive more food than it can use and assimilate, is to invite disaster and pave the way to physical bankruptcy. A knowledge of banking is valuable in any walk of life, and I feel that the most valuable advice I can give my readers is to study Nature's bookkeeping, as manifested in the human bank, and to see that the balance is strictly drawn between income and expenditure. The world will yet see the day when it will be considered a disgrace to be sick; but in the meantime, humanity suffers for lack of that important knowledge--knowledge of self.

Above all, cultivate the habit of happiness. Whatever else you may neglect, do not neglect that, for the happy habit is the greatest treasure that any individual can possess. Happiness depends largely upon physical conditions. With poor health, perfect happiness rarely exists; therefore it is your duty to be healthy, and the possession of health is in the majority of cases a matter of personal endeavor. But although the physical is important in health, yet the physical is dominated by the mental, and if you resolve to be happy, you can succeed. Commence this day, by saying to yourself, I am happy; I will be happy. Start out with the resolve that you will at least do some one thing to-day that will bring happiness to another, in the form of some simple service. Even if no such opportunity presents itself (although opportunities are never lacking), you can at least bestow cordial and cheerful greetings on those with whom you come in contact.

No surer road to personal happiness can be found than endeavoring to make others happy. If you find it difficult to be cheerful, there is more need to look to your surroundings. Read none but cheerful books; cultivate cheerful acquaintances. You will be amply repaid for your endeavors to cultivate the habit of happiness. From the standpoint of health, it is a profitable proceeding, for joy quickens the circulation. You can get the happiness habit if you wish to, and it is your duty to yourself and those around you to do so. If the clouds are lowering, do not give way to depression. Rouse yourself. Look for the rift in the clouds, disclosing the little patch of blue, and hope for the triumph of fair weather over foul. Even if you do not attain the degree of happiness you anticipated, you will find yourself improved, mentally, morally and physically. Get the habit, remembering that "a happy and contented mind is a continual feast."

And now, in conclusion, I would ask the reader to carefully consider the facts herein set forth relating to disease and its treatment, to weigh the testimony AGAINST the old system, and FOR the new, and let sober reason decide which of the two is the more rational. Bring the same dispassionate judgment to bear on this question that you would on a matter involving your financial welfare. It will amply repay you to do so, for the matter at stake is a weighty one. The preservation of health is a DUTY that each member of the human family owes to self and friends.

Without health, existence is as torpid and lifeless as vegetation without the sun. And yet it is frequently thrown away in thoughtless negligence, or in foolish experiments on our own strength: We let it perish without remembering its value, or waste it to show how much we have to spare. It is sometimes given up to levity and chance, and sometimes sold for the applause of jollity and looseness. Some there are, who inherit weak constitutions, and fall an easy prey to sickness; while others, who are neither thoughtless or naturally weak, invite disease through simple ignorance of the laws that govern their being. Owing to these manifold causes sickness is rife, and the medical profession has come to be regarded as an exceedingly lucrative one.

This would not be a matter so much to be deplored, if so-called "medical science" had kept pace with the other sciences; but the lamentable truth is that the practice of medicine (so far as healing value is concerned) has not advanced one jot since the days of Esculapius. Surgery has made wonderful strides, but medicine has stood still. True, they have increased the number of remedies, aye, a hundredfold, but the only result has been to complicate the system, without improving it.

What people need is fewer doctors, and more instruction in the art of preserving health.

Hygiene should form a part of our school curriculum. Children should be taught the mysteries of their own bodies, then the future generation would have little need of medical men--they would know what to do to regain their health, when assailed by sickness, instead of feeing a professional man to order them what to take.

My purpose in this work has been to show the people that they can, if they will, be their own physicians, and that in doing so, their chances of recovery are immeasurably greater--that the preservation of their health is in their own hands. The administering of drugs in sickness is illogical in its reasoning, unsound in its theory, and pernicious in its practice. Thoroughly cleansing the system by flushing the colon is a simple, common sense method of treatment, easy of application, thoroughly hygienic in theory, and, beyond all question, immensely beneficial in practice.

Thousands of grateful people can testify to its efficiency, frequently in cases where the "faculty" had abandoned all hope, and why? Because it assists Nature instead of thwarting it. The principal drawback under which the system has labored hitherto, has been the lack of perfect apparatus for the introduction of the cleansing stream, but I now have the satisfaction of introducing to the public a means for that purpose that leaves nothing to be desired. The J. B. L. Cascade is the most satisfactory and effective appliance for flushing the intestinal canal that has yet been invented.

It is the outcome of years of patient toil and thought, but the thoroughly satisfactory results obtained by it, and the enthusiastic encomiums lavished upon it by its beneficiaries are regarded by the inventor as an ample and commensurate reward (not wholly undeserved) for the mental labor involved in its successful evolution.

Its simplicity is such that it can be manipulated by any intelligent child, and its price, by comparison with its remedial virtues, is insignificant. With this perfected apparatus, and the J.B.L. antiseptic tonic, any parent can constitute himself the physician of his family, and by following the directions for the treatment of the various diseases described in this work, can successfully combat them-- and all at a trifling cost. But more than that, he can, by periodical use of it, so improve the physical condition of himself and family, that they will forget what sickness is, and rejoice in that exhilaration of spirit that only comes with perfect health.

My system of treatment is true in philosophy, in harmony with nature, and thoroughly rational in practice.

###

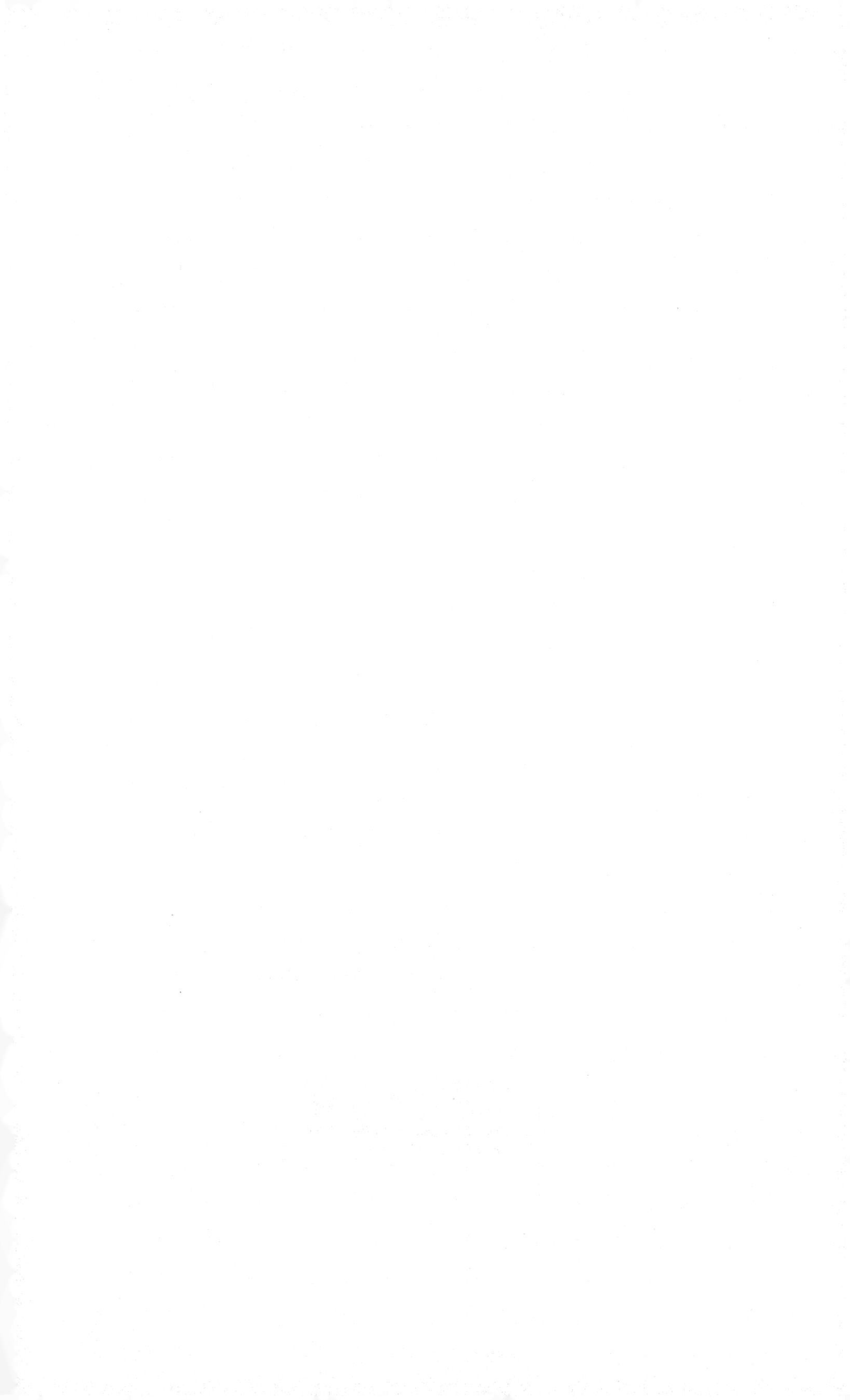

Made in the USA
Middletown, DE
09 January 2023

21767892R00086